LIVIN

...rnal-
...ked as
a BBC TV correspondent ...por... ...d the
world on wars, famines and disasters. She nas also
presented the main *Six O'clock News* on BBC1 and the
Today programme on Radio Four. She has written and
presented a number of investigative documentaries on
health and environmental issues. In more recent years
Triona has specialized in health-related journalism both
on TV and in print, writing articles for *The Times* and
Daily Mail. Triona is a patron of the Hughes Syndrome
Foundation. She lives in north London with her two
daughters, Tallulah and Aurora.

Overcoming Common Problems Series

For a full list of titles please contact
Sheldon Press, 1 Marylebone Road, London NW1 4DU

Overcoming Common Problems Series

Overcoming Common Problems Series

Overcoming Common Problems

Living with Hughes Syndrome

Triona Holden

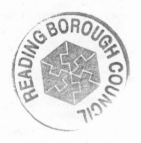

sheldon **PRESS**

Published in Great Britain in 2002 by
Sheldon Press
1 Marylebone Road
London NW1 4DU

British Library Cataloguing-in-Publication Data
A catalogue record for this book is available from the British Library

ISBN 0–85969–884–X

Typeset by Deltatype Limited, Birkenhead, Merseyside
Printed in Great Britain by Biddles Ltd
www.biddles.co.uk

Contents

To my daughters Tallulah and Aurora who helped me get through so much, and to all the courageous people who waived their anonymity to share their highly personal and moving stories in the hope of helping others

Foreword

Listen to the patient, for they are telling you the diagnosis.

This was the very first sentence I heard on my introductory ward round as a medical student at The Royal London Hospital. It has stuck with me ever since. I believe it should be the first lesson for every aspiring doctor – and not only doctors.

In reading the manuscript of this book, I was struck by the deft and sympathetic way Triona Holden has continued this tradition. Rarely have I read such a clear and sympathetic approach to a medical condition which at best is complex, at worst daunting.

Yet, as Ms Holden points out, this may come to be the commonest and most important of the so-called 'autoimmune' diseases. And it is still under-diagnosed.

Perhaps the simplest way to highlight this is to pose the question to the practising general doctor: 'Do you, in your practice, have patients with recurrent headache or migraine? Or with miscarriage? Or with unexpected thrombosis, for example deep vein thrombosis, or unexpectedly young patients suffering from memory loss, heart attacks or stroke? Or with odd neurological problems, perhaps regarded as "atypical multiple sclerosis". Or with chronic fatigue, aches and pains, or depression – none of which seem to fit into any clear pattern?'

Yes? Well, of course there are many possible diagnoses. But one of them could be Hughes syndrome, also known as 'antiphospholipid syndrome' (APS), or, more colloquially, as 'sticky blood' – a condition for which a cheap diagnostic blood test is available, and also treatment which can change the lives of many, many patients.

In 1983 we published the first of a series of articles in medical journals describing the syndrome in detail. One of the plus points of running large clinics is that with experience, you begin to 'spot' clinical patterns. Thus it was that there in my lupus (systemic lupus erythematosus, an autoimmune disease) clinic, currently with 2 500 patients on our list, I noticed a group of people with a distinct set of clinical features. These included thrombosis (blood clots), 'neurological' disease (especially strokes and headaches, but also movement disorder and memory loss), sometimes low platelet counts (platelets are blood cells necessary for clotting), skin livedo (a blotchy appearance of the veins), and the presence in the blood of tell-tale antibodies called 'antiphospholipid antibodies'.

On every ward round, we would discuss this complex group of patients. As so often happens in medicine, once you spot a clinical picture, the story grows and the number of cases increases – in this case, dramatically.

We pointed out two important clinical facts. First, that the condition could affect arteries as well as veins; second, and crucially, that the condition could occur in the *absence* of lupus – the so-called *primary* antiphospholipid syndrome.

I have gone on record as saying – and I believe this very strongly – that the primary antiphospholipid syndrome will come to be recognized as a more common condition than lupus, having an impact on conditions as disparate as migraine, pregnancy, fertility, neurological disorders (including memory loss) and arterial disease.

My colleagues and I worked very hard to set up 'standardized' blood tests, and to educate and bring together those interested in the subject. In 1984 we held the rather grandly named 'First International Conference' on the subject, in London. This was followed in 1986 by the second at St Thomas' Hospital. Since then the subject has taken off with an international conference every two years. The most recent, the ninth, was held in France and attracted 800 participants.

At the sixth international conference in Leuven, Belgium, my colleagues honoured me by naming the syndrome 'Hughes syndrome'.

For me this was an honour, and one which I acknowledge with pride. Some eponymous diseases are 'small print'; others comprise perhaps five or six cases. In this disease, in a series of papers between 1983 and 1985, we not only described a large number of patients in detail, but filled in much of the clinical picture. The strokes, memory loss, arterial disease, the 'primary' syndrome, pulmonary hypertension, the strong association with recurrent miscarriage, the livedo, the low platelet tendency, the spinal cord disease, were all carefully documented. But we also developed and standardized anticardiolipin testing. Although it would not have been my style to name the syndrome anything other than 'antiphospholipid syndrome', the 'Hughes syndrome' eponym gives me particular pleasure, because of the enormous amount of work that went into identifying the syndrome.

In this work, I pay tribute to four colleagues: Dr Nigel Harris and Dr Aziz Gharavi, and later, Dr Ron Asherson – all of whom gave their all to the work – and subsequently, Dr Munther Khamashta, who has done so much as my right-hand man to develop the research aspects of the syndrome, especially in the field of recurrent miscarriage.

Hughes syndrome is now established – though still not sufficiently widely recognized. That is why I believe that books such as Triona Holden's are *so* important. Cases that, in retrospect, are shiningly obvious to those of us steeped in the clinic, are still missed.

There are few more enjoyable and positive experiences than working with these patients. Back in 1983, in one of my earliest papers in the *British Medical Journal*, I wrote:

'. . . for those of us hardened to nihilism by years of study of various autoantibodies in systemic lupus erythematosus there is a rare sense of excitement at the implications of the associations now being reported'.

Dr Graham Hughes, MD FRCP
St Thomas' Hospital, London

Preface

I was working on an article for *The Times* when I first stumbled across the condition known as 'sticky blood'. The piece was about lupus, my interest fired by the fact that I suffer from this disease. I had been interviewing one of the world's leading specialists, Dr Graham Hughes. We were huddled in his Tardis-like office at St Thomas' Hospital in central London and I'd been grilling him for an hour or so. Things were going well as he is a consummate performer in front of journalists and had given me plenty of strong quotes. The interview was winding down and I was about to shove my notebook back in my bag when Dr Hughes began talking about 'antiphospholipid syndrome'. I must have looked dumbstruck by this mouthful because he quickly explained that it was a relatively new condition known in lay terms as 'sticky blood' and it would become the most common autoimmune disease of the century.

Instinctively I picked up my notebook again and began to scribble. After twenty years as a correspondent you develop a nose for what we call a 'cracking tale' and this sounded like just that.

With the calm of a man talking about the weather Dr Hughes described the syndrome that thickened the blood and thereby caused clots. It affected men and women, young and old alike. It attacked any part of the body at any time. 'Sticky blood' was responsible for a quarter of recurrent miscarriages and a fifth of strokes in young people. It was often mistaken for multiple sclerosis (MS) or early Alzheimer's. It caused deep vein thrombosis – including so called 'economy class syndrome' – memory loss, speech difficulties, headaches, fatigue and joint pains. It damaged major organs, made you blind or even killed you.

Another key concern was how many patients struggled for years to get a diagnosis and had often been mis-diagnosed, mainly as a result of medical ignorance about 'sticky blood'. At one recent clinic three people who'd been told they had MS were tested and told that in fact they had Hughes syndrome. The difference could not have been more profound: multiple sclerosis can consign the sufferer to what can be an appalling degenerative condition; the disease has varying degrees of severity but no matter how it affects someone the treatments available for the symptoms are limited and very expensive. On the other hand, there is a broad range of medications for 'sticky blood' which have been shown to be highly effective; these drugs are generally inexpensive and easily available, like aspirin, for example.

That was the good news about Hughes syndrome, the 'magic', as Dr Hughes would say. It was highly treatable with medication that thinned the blood, even something as mild as 'junior' (low-dose) aspirin would work. The cost was minimal, and there was an excellent chance that given the right monitoring a patient could live a normal life. The moving stories of the people in this book bear this out. Like the woman who was virtually blind for example, and after a few weeks of treatment got her eyesight back, or the former airline stewardess who found herself confined to a wheelchair, unable to control fierce spasms in her lower body, but after one week of treatment was walking with the help of sticks and is now striding up and down hospital corridors helping others in her situation by tirelessly devoting her time to the Hughes Syndrome Foundation.

Dr Hughes said that one area where they have had their greatest triumphs against this disease is in pregnancy. Women who had been through the agony of repeated miscarriages, some suffering twenty or more, had been given anticoagulants to thin their blood and had gone on to have healthy babies. For the first time I noticed the pictures that clung to the walls of Dr Hughes' office; they were mainly of mothers and children with beaming smiles. The pregnancy clinic showed a success rate that rose from under 20 per cent to over 75 per cent.

I am not known for being lost for words but there was a moment when my mouth fell open and I was silent. The weight of what I had heard was staggering. Here we had a new condition that was common but as yet seriously under-diagnosed. It touched on every area of medicine and affected a significant slice of the population – not just of Britain, where it was first identified – but of all over the world. A plethora of questions came to mind but the most pressing was: why hadn't I heard of Hughes syndrome?

One reason could have been that it is still a 'new' disease, first identified by Dr Hughes in the early 1980s. Another relates to the age-old issue of funding. To do lots of research or have the staff and time to get the message across takes money, a commodity that is not in large supply in this field of medicine in the UK. Those involved in treating patients are too busy doing just that and don't have time to worry about writing press releases and publicity. It is rather like HIV or lupus, it has taken time to recognize these new conditions, and to get the message out.

As a sufferer of lupus I know first-hand how difficult it is to cope with having an autoimmune disease where the range of symptoms is broad and diverse. The biggest hurdle is the first – namely getting the diagnosis. When I became ill, before we had a name for the disease, I had so many things wrong with me that I wrestled with the fear I was going mad. I tried to ignore my symptoms for as long as I could, hoping they would go away. Not an easy task when I could no longer pick up my children for a cuddle without experiencing excruciating pain in my shoulders and chest and muscle weakness in my arms. Or when a simple task such as getting up the stairs left me shuffling on my bottom taking one step at a time as my aching hip and knee joints just wouldn't do as they were told. My feet were so numb that I could put them in scalding water without feeling it. Typing no longer came automatically, my mind had to guide the frozen fingers across the keys. Worst of all was the fatigue. For someone who lived on her energy waking up to a flat battery was as good as a prison sentence. Some days I would lie in bed and feel as though I had an elephant sitting on me. I couldn't move.

And all the time in my head I doubted this was really happening to me. As I lay prone in my bed listening to my 12-year-old getting the 7-year-old ready for school because 'mummy wasn't well', I would tell myself off for slacking. In my head I would see all the jobs I had to get on with, work out the agenda for the day. The trouble was that my body didn't respond to the call for action.

How could it be that every part of me was involved? From my eyes to the tips of my toes, with lots in between. I was embarrassed to tell the whole story to my consultant. The monologue went on and on, the student doctors would raise their eyebrows – impressed by such a catalogue of illness. In the end I would do a summary of symptoms on my laptop, and hand him a printed copy. It took two years to get a diagnosis and in that time I had a plethora of tests. They took armfuls of blood, a biopsy of my lip, I was irradiated, X-rayed, warmed up and cooled down. I felt like a laboratory animal but I was glad of any efforts made to give my illness a name. It sounds odd but when I was eventually diagnosed as having a form of systemic lupus erythematosus (SLE) I actually felt delighted – not because I had an incurable and potentially life-threatening disease but because at long last I had a name, and that meant I could find out more about the illness, and fight it.

As with lupus, getting a diagnosis for Hughes syndrome is notoriously difficult. The campaign to improve awareness of SLE has been working hard for over a decade. 'Sticky blood' is still virtually under wraps on this front. This means there is limited information available in the public domain so far. Trawl through bookshops and you are likely to come out empty handed. If you look on the internet there are some sites that are helpful: the Hughes Syndrome Foundation is one and you can order the book written by Dr Hughes called *A Patient's Guide*, which gives a excellent explanation of the disease from a medical perspective. But if you are like me, you always want more, you want to hear from fellow sufferers so you can compare notes. That is why this book is built up around a core of people who have 'sticky blood' and are happy to tell their stories. Perhaps what they went through rings a bell and might prompt others to put the pieces of the jigsaw together. That would bring them one step closer to getting some answers and stopping this disease from doing any more damage.

After hearing about 'sticky blood' from Dr Hughes I wrote a piece for *The Times* which triggered off a staggering response from readers who jammed the switchboard at the clinic in St Thomas' and generated more than 70 000 'hits' on the Hughes Syndrome Foundation website in a matter of days. I couldn't help but feel I was just scratching the surface and there was a pressing need to make more information available to the public at large. Hence this book.

When you find you have a major illness you unwillingly and unwittingly join a club. Only fellow members can understand the dreadful reality of what you are going through. As a fully paid up member I feel qualified to know something of what it is you need. I am a journalist not a doctor so I approach the subject from the point of view of the lay person. What I have tried to do is plough through the medical jargon, sift out the facts and present them to you so that they are easily understood. It is important to remember you are not alone, that is why so many patients have happily agreed to talk openly in this book about what happened to them. As 'club' members they know how lonely and depressing illness can be. The disease is common, it just so happens that it is early days and you are having to do more research than those who follow in your footsteps. It is also crucial you hang onto the knowledge that there is plenty you can do about this disease if you test positive for it. The key is to get the diagnosis; to do that you need to know what to look for, who to insist on seeing and what tests and treatment you might require. I hope this book gives you the information, support and encouragement you need to fight 'sticky blood'.

Triona Holden, London, 2002

1

'Know the Enemy'

In a war one of the most effective weapons you can have is 'intelligence'; it is vital to have as much information about the enemy as possible. The same scenario applies to any illness. This is particularly true with 'sticky blood'. Although in the next decade most people will have heard of this condition, at the moment it is relatively new and to-date awareness is frustratingly poor in the general public and worst of all within the medical profession. It is therefore wise to arm yourself with as much information as you can, that way you improve your chances of getting in front of the right experts and being given the treatment that could be life-saving. It is possible that you will end up knowing more than some of the doctors who examine you.

First things first. Let's tackle the name of this condition. Originally it was called 'antiphospholipid syndrome' or 'APS', and in many areas of the world like the USA this name is still commonly used. I know it's a mouthful and probably means nothing at all to you unless you are medically trained in some way. I will go into what antiphospholipid antibodies are later. For now, I would like to give you two other much more user-friendly names that feature throughout this book. The condition was renamed a few years ago in honour of the renowned British physician Dr Graham Hughes, who first identified this illness, so it changed from 'antiphospholipid syndrome' to 'Hughes syndrome'. The other name is 'sticky blood'. This way of referring to the disease was coined by the media, it is not scientific, nor is it completely accurate but it cleverly describes what the condition actually does. It is also easy to remember and not as hard to spell as antiphospholipid!

The next step is to get an idea of what the disease is and how it works. The battleground is within your own body. The enemy is the very mechanism that would normally protect you, namely your immune system. Hughes syndrome is diverse and fickle, it is a condition that recognizes few medical boundaries. This is because of how it works. In simple terms the immune system turns in on itself and becomes overactive. The body is fighting imaginary intruders and in the process the blood becomes thicker and is therefore more

1

likely to clot. As blood is involved in every part of the body the disease has free access to wherever it decides to target. It can strike anyone regardless of sex or age. Patients range from toddlers suffering strokes to pensioners having clots in their legs. It can affect any part of the body at any time for no apparent reason. There is no limit to the range of the disease: sufferers can have mild symptoms and live a relatively normal life or they can be so ill they are confined to bed or wheelchair. In the worst cases Hughes syndrome can be fatal. The disease can mimic other illnesses and that makes it difficult to diagnose. For instance, doctors working in this field are finding a significant number of patients being referred to them who have been told they are probably in the early stages of multiple sclerosis. When they are given the simple blood test for 'sticky blood' it has come back positive. The difference could not be more profound: MS can be a progressively and permanently debilitating disease whereas the symptoms of Hughes syndrome are highly treatable and can be controlled effectively. A later chapter in this book deals with MS and this syndrome.

Clearly getting a diagnosis is difficult because of the varied symptoms, and doctors won't find Hughes syndrome if they are not looking for it. Anyone who has been suffering for months and possibly years dreads seeing his or her doctor and hearing 'I'm afraid we just don't know'. Those few words can be devastating if you are the one left in the dark. You begin to wonder whether or not you have been imagining all those ailments, you worry that perhaps you are behaving like a hypochondriac. I have interviewed many sufferers who had been told that they were having a hysterical reaction and given antidepressants. Hopefully reading this book will help convince some people that they are not losing their marbles, they are just unwell.

Hughes syndrome is not a rare condition, it is responsible for a quarter of all recurrent miscarriages and one in five strokes in people under 40 in Britain. The 'word' is getting out as more information becomes available, doctors in particular are reading up on 'sticky blood'. Dr Hughes is quite clear on the question of how common it is: 'I believe that this syndrome will become the most diagnosed autoimmune disease of the twenty-first century, more prevalent than rheumatoid arthritis, lupus, MS or ME.'

It is also possible that 1 in 200 of people in high-risk groups would prove positive for Hughes syndrome. Worldwide that is a staggering number, it is like a disaster waiting to happen.

If you are reading this book it means you are likely to have heard of 'sticky blood' or Hughes syndrome. It also means you suspect or know that you or someone close to you has this condition. You will probably be desperately searching for more information and have found there is precious little available at the moment. This book should provide answers to your questions and if not the last section in the book (p. 89) will help direct you to other sources of information.

What do you look out for? Each patient is different but there are a number of major symptoms that are danger signs:

- Blood clots in the veins or arteries.
- Miscarriage for the second or third time. Doctors term this 'recurrent miscarriage' and will investigate only then. However, Dr Hughes believes tests should be done after just one late (after 12 weeks' gestation) miscarriage.
- Stroke, especially under 40 years.
- Memory loss, speech difficulties, symptoms of early Alzheimer's disease.
- Headaches, migraine and fits.
- Pins-and-needles, difficulty with balance or vision, symptoms associated with multiple sclerosis.
- Extreme fatigue.
- Muscle pains and cramp.
- Blotchy skin – known by doctors as *livedo reticularis*, where the blood vessels can be seen under the skin.
- Low platelet (blood cells responsible for clotting) count that can lead to bruising.

If a doctor suspects you might have Hughes syndrome there are two simple blood tests that are available worldwide and are inexpensive to carry out. The first test is for anticardiolipin antibodies, commonly referred to as aCL. The second has a confusing name, lupus anticoagulant, or LA, but this test has nothing to do with lupus. The 'science' of it is that normally the body has its own natural protection against too much clotting, but if you have Hughes syndrome it means your immune system has produced proteins, or antibodies, that make the blood far more sticky than normal and therefore more liable to clot. These antibodies alter the shape of the platelets (the blood cells responsible for clotting) and the walls of the blood vessels, and this in turn affects the free flow of the blood.

Why does this happen? At the moment no one is very sure what lies behind Hughes syndrome. There is some evidence there could be a genetic link, and some of the contributors in this book are convinced 'sticky blood' has run in their family undetected for generations. It is frustrating not to be able to point to a cause and say 'there, that's the culprit' but as with many autoimmune conditions things just aren't that straightforward.

People often ask if it has to do with stress. There is no simple answer to that. Dr Hughes has found that there does seem to be a link but there is no research to back this up. In talking to patients it is quite clear that they often believe there is a direct connection between something major happening in their lives and a flare-up of the disease. Some find that even when they are on medication an increase in stress, such as pressures at work or the break-up of a relationship, will act as a trigger for the symptoms to return. It is also common sense that a terrible event in your life, like losing your job or the end of your marriage, will affect your health, especially if it is already erratic.

There is also evidence that a viral infection might trigger 'sticky blood'. Patients have reported suffering first of all with a sore throat or flu and then going on to have more symptoms. Is diet a factor? No one knows; the current wisdom is the same for virtually any illness – eat a balanced diet and take regular exercise. You might want to quiz other members of the family, or check your family history, see if older generations suffered thrombosis, strokes, recurrent miscarriages, severe headaches or even growing pains. It is possible the clues you need to trace your illness are staring out at you from your family tree.

Some patients turn to alternative medicines, and this is discussed later (see p. 87), but their effectiveness is hard to judge. Mainstream medical treatment has much to offer: there is plenty of evidence that it works and can improve things within days if not hours, often without nasty side-effects. Think of it logically, if you have thick blood the answer must be to thin it, it sounds so simple and in a way it is. The pharmaceutical industry has developed a whole range of drugs known as 'anticoagulants' or blood thinners. These include warfarin and heparin and, most common of all, aspirin. There can be side-effects but this varies with each individual. New versions of these drugs are being developed all the time.

Once a patient is diagnosed as having Hughes syndrome, doctors will keep a close eye on his/her blood, monitoring what is known as the INR (international normalized ratio). This, in other words, is a way of checking if the blood falls within what is regarded as a normal blood thickness. The test for this is most often carried out at the local hospital or doctor's surgery, although home test kits are available. Even a tiny fluctuation in the INR can result in the return of symptoms such as slurred speech, headaches, visual disturbance, blood clot and mini-strokes. Many patients who have known their condition for years have become such experts at recognizing the warning signs that they get help before they become dangerously ill again.

2
Clots

Have you ever had a blood clot? It doesn't matter where, when or how serious it was. What matters is the fact that you have suffered from a thrombosis, the medical term for a stationary blood clot. If the answer is 'Yes' then it is possible that your blood is thicker than it ought to be. This puts you at risk of having further, possibly more serious, clots. As part of your treatment, you can also insist on being checked for Hughes syndrome. Details of the blood tests are in Chapter 13.

The commonest areas affected by blood clots in the veins are the legs (unusually in the deep veins) and arms, but they can also affect smaller veins in organs such as the kidney, liver and eyes. One of the greatest dangers with a clot is that it might break up and travel to another part of the body, such as the heart, brain or lungs. In any of these areas a clot can prove fatal. At first patients may suffer minor clots, and these are regarded as an early warning.

Another aspect of clotting in Hughes syndrome is that, unlike other clotting disorders, it can also cause thrombosis in the arteries. This type of clot, which may affect major organs like the brain and the heart, can have much more severe consequences. An arterial clot can lead to what are known as TIAs (transient ischaemic attacks) in the brain (when the brain is momentarily deprived of oxygen) or strokes, which can result in permanent memory loss, speech difficulties, headaches and seizures. A thrombosis in an artery can also lead to an angina or heart attack.

The presence of a clot is the single most dramatic sign that someone might be suffering from Hughes syndrome. A lot has been written in recent years about deep vein thrombosis (DVT) – a blood clot (thrombus) lodged in one of the deep veins of the leg. The number of people becoming ill or even dying after travelling by plane pushed DVT into the spotlight. The condition was dubbed 'economy class syndrome' by the media because it was widely thought that cramped conditions in the cabin of an aircraft contributed to or caused a blood clot. It took the tragic deaths of a number of otherwise healthy young passengers to create enough pressure on governments and airlines to look into cabin safety.

Studies are under way into whether economy class syndrome is a reality or simply a figment of an overexcited press. The airlines themselves are funding some of that research; it makes good business sense to be seen to be doing something other than issuing vague warnings and support stockings. Perhaps it is surprising then that major airlines have chosen to ignore compelling evidence that a good percentage of these DVTs are likely to be the result of a person having 'sticky blood', a condition that is exacerbated by the cramped conditions in a pressurized aircraft cabin but not caused by them. The better news is that the British government has said a review of cabin safety would include a look at DVT and 'sticky blood'.

Dr Hughes is firmly of the belief that if those people who suffered a DVT after being on a plane were tested for 'sticky blood' a significant percentage of them would prove to be positive, possibly as many as one in four. He has seen a considerable number of patients who have had clots during or after flights, and they all tested positive for Hughes syndrome. To date, research into links between DVT and 'sticky blood' has been limited; in time though as more cases of this kind come to light it will be possible to establish a firm connection. For passengers this would be great news. It would give them a chance of preventing DVT or getting treated quickly if they suffered one during or after a flight. Dr Hughes wants to see passengers given a simple questionnaire with their ticket which would assess how at risk they were. It would ask seven questions:

- Have you ever suffered a blood clot?
- Do you have recurrent migraine or severe headaches?
- Are your fingers and toes numb?
- Is there a family history of autoimmune disease?
- Have you had two or more miscarriages?
- Do you suffer memory loss or speech difficulties?
- Have you had treatment for poor circulation?

If a person answers 'Yes' to any of these questions then there is an increased likelihood he or she could have Hughes syndrome, and so should be screened for 'sticky blood'. Identifying those who are at risk of having DVT will save lives and be effective in terms of preventing clots.

Dr Jenny Dautlich

Dr Jenny Dautlich knew she suffered from an autoimmune

disorder when she boarded a flight from London to New York three years ago. She had suffered a deep vein thrombosis 13 years before and had been treated with anticoagulants ever since. As she was taking the medication it wasn't unreasonable for her to feel safe as she buckled her seatbelt ready for the journey. Jenny, who is originally from Ecuador, had moved to England years before to do her postgraduate training in medicine. She suffered a blood clot in her left leg when she was 28. 'I was perfectly healthy and then I got this terrible pain in my left leg. It was a large clot and they decided to remove it. After that I was put on warfarin to thin my blood'.

The interim years had been unremarkable healthwise. In fact Jenny had become frustrated with having to stay on medication when she felt well. She went to the Royal Free Hospital in north London to have tests so she could stop taking the warfarin. The results were disappointing for her, 'I didn't want to be on warfarin any more but the blood tests showed I had to continue taking anticoagulants. The doctors there thought I had lupus but I was a borderline case; there was no mention of Hughes syndrome as I believe no one had heard of it.'

Jenny was 41 when she boarded the plane to the USA. She was on warfarin but her INR (international normalized ratio) was very low that day – 1.3 when it was normally 3.0–4.0. Jenny says the flight departure was brought forward: 'They changed the times of my flight, I would have taken more warfarin if I had had more time.' It is unclear whether that would have made any difference to the near fatal events that followed.

During the flight Jenny was fine, a little tired but she put that down to the usual fatigue that accompanies travel: 'I had been told to drink lots of water and take as much exercise as I could. I did both these things. I felt tired but nothing else.'

It was the next day at her aunt's house in New York that she began to feel very unwell. She felt as though her head was about to explode, the pain was devastating. Jenny was dizzy and began vomiting.' I was having a bad headache, it was very strong. As a doctor I knew I was in trouble, I knew I was very unwell but I was so confused and in such pain that it was difficult for me to fully understand what was happening. My brother-in-law is a doctor and the family called him. He told them to take me to hospital as quickly as possible.' Jenny's sister called a cab; luckily there was a large hospital nearby.

'I remember being frustrated because in the emergency area the nurse was more concerned with writing down my details than checking my blood pressure. When she did get around to doing my blood pressure was dangerously low; it was then that the alarm bells started ringing. I asked to see a doctor as I was one and felt I could move things along but the nurse didn't listen.

'I knew in my heart that I was very sick. I am a Christian so I began praying, then I took off my rings and my watch and gave them to my sister, I thought I was going to die. As they took me to another room I told my sister not to cry and promised that I would be back, I just wasn't sure when. In truth I didn't know if I could keep that promise. After that I fell into a coma.'

Jenny suffered a massive heart attack as well as a DVT. Once at the hospital, whilst she was being treated for the heart attack she suffered a series of strokes. When she came round her right side was paralysed. She could not see or speak, her right arm and leg were frozen.

Blood tests were done to see what might be wrong. Jenny says they told her she might have antiphospholipid syndrome, the original name for Hughes syndrome. 'I had never heard of it and there wasn't much information available so I was in the dark, I didn't know what it meant.' In Jenny's case it very nearly meant death. But she pulled through and gradually recovered some of her health.

When Jenny was well enough she returned to England with her husband Wilfred. Jenny was taking anticoagulant medication to prevent a recurrence of DVT. Since the stroke Jenny has worked hard to get back some of what she lost. 'My right arm is still paralysed but I am learning to write again, and I have seen a speech therapist. These days I can read again but I still only have partial vision in my left eye.' Jenny has regained much of her speech. She still has flares which are controlled by anticoagulants. Determined to get on with her life Jenny is currently training in public health and wants to work within the NHS.

There are a number of recognized factors that contribute to a deep vein thrombosis: smoking, prolonged immobility and the contraceptive pill are a few of them. If a woman has Hughes syndrome the chances of a DVT during pregnancy are increased as the blood becomes naturally stickier, and once a person has suffered one DVT the chances are that he or she will go on to have further episodes.

Hilary Swarbrick

It was when Hilary Swarbrick was pregnant with her son in 1986 that she had her first clot in her leg. Treatment dealt with the clot but her pregnancy was dogged by severe migraine attacks. Hilary had a history of these headaches as well as circulation problems, varicose veins and a discoloration of her feet.

'In 1989 I developed a DVT in my right leg and spent a week in hospital on an intravenous heparin drip. When I was discharged I was prescribed warfarin for three months and told that the probable cause of the clot was the contraceptive pill I had been taking.'

For the next five years Hilary found she had more symptoms without knowing what was wrong. She had bouts of phlebitis – a painful condition where veins (usually in the legs) become inflamed, often leading to clots. The migraine persisted, she also had pain in her legs and chronic fatigue. Hilary was pregnant with her second child and at nine weeks developed another clot in her right leg. She was given heparin injections and tested for lupus and Hughes syndrome. The result showed she had antiphospholipid antibodies. During her 30-week antenatal appointment the doctor couldn't find the baby's heartbeat. A scan confirmed Hilary's worst fears – her baby had died. She gave birth to Liam two days later. She was devastated. And things got worse. As they waited for their baby's body to be returned after a post-mortem she developed another DVT. After Liam's funeral she was admitted to hospital. She later learnt that Liam had died because clots had formed in her placenta, starving him of food and oxygen.

After reading an article on the work at St Thomas' Hospital, Hilary saw Dr Hughes. 'After being diagnosed with Hughes I felt so isolated and was in desperate need of information about my condition. I wanted to talk to someone who understood what I was going through but there was little out there for people like me. To save others going through the despair that I had, I decided to start a support line. On 28 January 1996 with the help of my health visitor, Ronnie Bray, I started the Hughes Syndrome Foundation.'

Hilary saw Dr Munther Khamashta at St Thomas', she attended his pregnancy clinic for those with Hughes syndrome. 'In January 1997 I became pregnant and this time I was closely monitored by my GP, the local hospital and St Thomas'. I attended a clinic regularly for blood tests, check-ups and Doppler blood flow scans. Although success wasn't guaranteed, I always came away from Dr Hughes' clinic with a sense of optimism. On the 26 September I gave birth to a healthy baby girl by Caesarean section.'

Hilary still has bouts of chronic tiredness, joint pain and circulatory problems but since starting the warfarin she no longer has migraine attacks or DVTs.

Hélène Heilpern

Travel is a big part of Hélène Heilpern's life. She and her husband have a home in London and the south of France so they are always on the move.

Over the years Hélène was also used to travelling further afield to visit a close friend in Sri Lanka; the numerous long haul flights had no effect, that is until 2001.

'I had been on umpteen flights to Sri Lanka. My friend had lived there for three years and I would see her often, her husband is in the diplomatic service so I would go to keep her company or on holiday. I am godmother to her three children.

'I never had a problem with the journey until my trip last year. I had a few seats together so I managed to lie down and sleep for most of the flight, I felt absolutely fine. My friend picked me up at the airport and the next day we travelled to the seaside with the children. It was about five days after the flight that my left leg began to swell. I thought I had been bitten by something so I wasn't too fussed about it. But the swelling increased. Two days later I saw a doctor in the hospital who diagnosed cellulitis (a bacterial infection of the skin). He gave me some antibiotics and a stocking to wear but it was far too tight as by now the swelling was so bad my leg was three times its normal size.

'The following week I was due to fly home, the doctor said that I would be fine, but by then I was having difficulty walking because my leg was so bad. I needed a wheelchair at the airport. When I got back to the UK I was due to fly to Nice, France the next day to join my husband. I felt so unwell that my mother came to help me pack.

'When I got to Nice I had to walk to the customs' hall as they didn't have a wheelchair, it was agony. They even called my husband in to help me clear customs. He was angry with me for making the journey.

'The next day I saw a general physician. Within minutes he had called an ambulance and I was on my way to hospital. I was admitted to the intensive care unit. They did an ultrasound and found six clots in my leg.'

Hélène had no idea what danger she had been in, she still thought she was suffering from a bacterial infection, not deep vein thrombosis. The French doctors treated her with strong anticoagulants to deal with the clots. This seemed to work well and after a few days they gave her the all-clear to go home.

'On the day I was due to leave hospital I had a terrible pain in my lower abdomen, they did some tests and found there were cysts on my ovaries that were bleeding because of the anticoagulants. They had to operate to stop the bleeding. Fortunately the operation was a success and I was allowed home.

'These days I am on warfarin all the time and when I fly I use support stockings.'

Before this episode, Hélène knew she had lupus. She was diagnosed when she was just 20 years old, 27 years before the DVTs. She had just got married and was trying to study at university to become a dietician. Hélène developed several odd symptoms: 'I was just a complete mess. I couldn't control my body. My legs and arms would move around, so would my tongue. I wouldn't speak to anyone because when I did try to talk all that would come out was gibberish. I didn't speak to anyone for a month; I was so frightened by having no control. They put me on a massive dose of steroids. Then a doctor at my local hospital said he knew of a man "who seemed to deal with this kind of disease". So I went to see Dr Hughes, and it is a tribute to him that I was well for 27 years before I had the clots.'

Hélène was diagnosed as having Hughes syndrome in 2001 and she is being treated with anticoagulants. It now seems likely that she had a stroke when she was 20, although there is no way of knowing for sure. It is also likely that she developed Hughes syndrome over the years, as well as having lupus. There are a growing number of cases like Hélène's where a person who originally tested negative for 'sticky blood' but positive for lupus has gone on to test positive for the antiphospholipid antibodies in subsequent years. It does not work the other way round though: if you have Hughes syndrome you are very unlikely to go on to have lupus.

3
Baby Blues

Any woman who has suffered a miscarriage will know what a lonely and devastating experience it can be. It is often made worse by the fact that those around her, including her doctor, will tell her not to worry and to try conceiving again as soon as her health allows. From a woman's point of view miscarriage can seem like one of the harshest and most unsympathetic areas of medicine. After losing one pregnancy the current medical wisdom is that this is common and in general nothing to worry about, especially if it is early on. Losing a second baby is not so common but also not something that would cause undue concern. It is only when a woman has had three miscarriages that the alarm bells start to ring and the medical machine kicks into action. A woman is then told she suffers from 'recurrent miscarriage', and with that the tests and investigations begin.

This system takes little account of how distressing even one miscarriage can be for a woman or couple wanting to start a family. The trauma of having lost three or more babies is hard to imagine if it hasn't happened to you. It is a painful situation often compounded by the apparent disregard for the first two miscarriages. A considerable number of women I have spoken to for this book felt more could have been done sooner. They were convinced there was an underlying problem that was not being addressed. They struggled to be heard by their doctors and felt they were only taken seriously after they had suffered three miscarriages; in some cases that meant years of uncertainty, not knowing what was wrong. But what has this got to do with 'sticky blood'? Miscarriage is one of the main clues that a woman might be suffering from Hughes syndrome. One in four cases of recurrent miscarriage is due to this condition. Dr Hughes is of the view that women should be tested for antiphospholipid antibodies after just one miscarriage, or the blood test should be part of routine antenatal screening. The test could be an early indicator that a woman needs special treatment to have a successful pregnancy, hopefully saving her the trauma of repeated miscarriage.

Mr Anthony Kenney, gynaecologist to the Duchess of York, says work in this field is groundbreaking. 'The discovery that Hughes syndrome affects so many pregnant women is the most significant development in obstetrics in 20 years. The implications for patients are tremendous – it means we can help prevent repeated miscarriage. This syndrome can cause repeated miscarriage in the middle three months of pregnancy – which is sad as the baby looks like a baby by then. It can also cause stillbirth, and – perhaps most devastating of all – premature labour, where up to 50 per cent of babies born as early as 25 weeks could suffer a range of complications such as blindness, deafness, paralysis and brain damage. So the significance of this is considerable. This work has given us more insight and has had an enormous impact on the lives of those struggling to start a family.'

Many women can have the antiphospholipid antibody prior to pregnancy without knowing anything is wrong. It is only when they become pregnant that the condition makes its presence felt. When a woman is carrying a baby her blood naturally becomes slightly more viscous or thick. So someone who also has 'sticky blood' is much more likely to have problems carrying the foetus to full term. One simple explanation for what happens is that the capillaries to the foetus from the placenta, which are fine and delicate, become blocked as clots prevent the blood (and so food and oxygen) getting to the foetus. Gradually the placenta withers, and the foetus fails to thrive and is aborted.

If the syndrome has been diagnosed there is plenty that can be done to help. The drugs available are very effective and can be as mild as junior aspirin. In later pregnancy women who are at risk are watched closely. The use of a Doppler monitor means doctors can keep an eye on the blood supply to the foetus. If the pulse wave begins to weaken or if there is a sign that there is a reversal of blood flow then an emergency Caesarean section can be performed.

The success rate at the pregnancy clinic at St Thomas' is staggering, rising from under 20 per cent to over 75 per cent. Some of the women patients have had 13 or more miscarriages; one lady had 20 plus. They were all women determined to succeed. The babies and toddlers at the clinic are a testament to the courage of these women and their families, and of course those running the show like Dr Munther Khamashta. The great thing is that for many of them there is a happy ending, or should I say beginning.

Sharon Montgomery

One woman whose bravery shines out is Sharon Montgomery. She was diagnosed with lupus when she was 20 years old. This was only after her GP at the time had dismissed her on a number of occasions saying the symptoms were in her head. She had joint pains, shortness of breath, severe coughing. With her father's help she saw a consultant rheumatologist who immediately admitted her to hospital; her heart had become enlarged and her kidneys were failing. With the right medication she pulled through but was in a wheelchair for months. She recovered well and married Adrian the following year. Sharon became pregnant, but sadly she miscarried early on.

'Four years later I became pregnant again. I was delighted but anxious. My fears were confirmed when I miscarried at eight weeks. I was referred to St Thomas' where more tests were carried out.'

Sharon became pregnant again and this time gave birth to a baby girl. But things were not right, Maxine was very premature and weighed only 1 lb (0.5 kg). She was a fighter but the odds were stacked against her and she died after three months.

The fact that she had given birth to a live baby gave Sharon and her husband hope that despite the difficulties they could make their dream of starting a family come true. Sharon had two more miscarriages and then gave birth to a baby boy, Matthew. He was born at 26 weeks and weighed $1\frac{1}{2}$ lb (0.7 kg). Tragedy struck again and baby Matthew died after only four days. To make matters even worse Sharon was acutely ill after the birth and had been rushed to the intensive care unit. She only saw Matthew once.

'I remember lying there and thinking how awful that it had happened again. I was devastated. I felt so ill, and I couldn't help wondering why this kept happening to me. But it was worst for Adrian, he had to rush between Matthew and myself as we were in two different hospital wards. He tried his best to keep a check on both of us to make sure we were stable and he hoped we were recovering. He was so worried about us, it was such a terrible time for him. Words cannot describe the pain when Matthew died, Adrian felt he never wanted to go through it all again. I could understand his feelings.'

Eighteen months later the couple changed their minds; they

decided to have one last try to start the family they longed for. Because they had come so close it was felt there was a good chance of success. Under the guidance of Dr Hughes, Sharon was given daily injections of heparin and had a weekly scan. She was admitted to hospital early and was cared for by a special midwifery team. At 32 weeks Sharon started to have problems with blood flow and blood pressure. Her baby was delivered by Caesarean section. Benedict Ashley weighed in at 3 lb (1.5 kg). Benedict was nicknamed 'Bam Bam' on the special care unit because his initials were BAM – but they could just as easily have been referring to his will to live. Benedict might have been small but he was strong. Sharon and Adrian's last gamble on having a child had paid off. 'We went through so much in those years of trying for a child and we came close to abandoning the whole thing. I am so glad we didn't. Benedict brings us such joy, he is now seven years old and so full of life.'

For Sharon and her husband Adrian the pain of 13 years of loss has melted away. 'When I look at Benedict I feel such joy, he loves his school and enjoys music and dance. I can't imagine life without him.'

Angela Steward

Angela Steward, a former product manager for the food manufacturers Chivers Hartley, was devastated when she was told her chances of having a baby were virtually nil. Angela, who's 31 and lives in Cambridgeshire, had suffered seven miscarriages. She was diagnosed as having Hughes syndrome. Despite a diagnosis after her third miscarriage the treatment Angela was given didn't help. It was only through sheer determination that she found her way to Dr Hughes and the team at St Thomas' and got the medication that helped turn her dream of becoming a mother into a reality.

'When my little girl arrived I couldn't stop crying. They were tears of utter joy. She was the miracle that I had longed for. I called her Jade because I read in a book that it meant "a mother's most precious gift" and she was certainly that to me.

'I had been trying for nine years to have a child, I had lost seven babies. I decided I would have one last try. I couldn't keep putting my husband, David, and myself through the trauma of it all.

'We married young, when we were both 20. It was about three years after that we decided the time was right to have children. It's a cruel irony that I spent so much time worrying that I might have become pregnant by mistake; it never occurred to me that I might not be able to have children when I decided I wanted them.

'I remember being so thrilled when I was first pregnant. It was my Mum and Dad's 25th wedding anniversary party. My Dad announced it to everyone there and he was beaming. Obviously we were too. Shortly after that I lost the baby. One of the hardest things was having to tell all these people that I wasn't pregnant any more.

'I had gone for my scan, my Nan came with me. I was so pleased she did because the baby had died at about ten-and-a-half weeks but the womb had kept on growing. It was awful.

'I left it a good year before trying again. But the same thing happened, that was disappointing and it was even worse because they told me that until a woman has had three miscarriages they wouldn't do any investigative work. I thought that I would get pregnant quite quickly this time because if there was a problem I wanted them to find out what it was.

'I did think a lot about what was wrong with me but the medical profession said it was just the law of averages and it was the sort of thing that happened all the time. What can you do when they say that? You have to trust that they know better than you do. I had the third miscarriage and they started to do some tests. I had other hints that something was wrong. I was having symptoms like terrible blinding headaches. My arms and legs were stiff and painful as well. I was only 26 but I felt like an old woman. I would say this to my doctor and I was sure that he thought I was a hypochondriac.

'It was a doctor in Cambridge who brought to light that I might have a condition called Hughes syndrome, which is also known as 'sticky blood'. A blood test confirmed this and I was put on injections of heparin and a daily dose of aspirin. I was desperate to know more but there wasn't much information available.

'I was sent to a number of specialists, including a haematologist and a neurologist. The main consultant was a rheumatologist. Then I got pregnant again and my case was sent back to my obstetrician. It was so confusing and I felt so out of control, like I was being pushed around and nobody was really helping me. I lost the baby after ten weeks of pregnancy. I went on to have yet another miscarriage, my fifth. I was devastated and the pressure on us as a couple was dreadful. The whole thing was destroying our marriage. I felt as though I was a failure as a woman, that David should find a partner who could give him children. It was such a hard time for both of us.

'Then I read an article in the *Daily Mail*'s 'Good Health' section, this was in December 1997. It was a report about a woman called Sharon Kelly who had the same condition as me. The treatment she had been on had helped her have a baby. I thought "Right, I'm going to look into this further". The article mentioned the team at St Thomas' Hospital in London. I knew that I had to get to see them as they were specialists in this field. I didn't want to be fobbed off again.

'I started phoning St Thomas' and I somehow got through to one of the leading doctors at the clinic, a lady called Dr Beverley Hunt, a consultant haematologist working in the Louise Coote Lupus Clinic. I was so lucky to speak to her, she was a remarkable person. She said it would be no problem getting an appointment, all I needed was a referral, but that proved difficult. There was so much red tape. I decided it was pointless going to the doctors to get what I wanted so I went to the people who held the purse strings, Cambridgeshire Health Authority. I was on their back constantly, phoning them all the time and nagging for a referral.

'At last it did come through and I got the appointment at St Thomas'. Even then there were problems, as my notes from Cambridge never arrived. So in the end the team at St Thomas' did all the basic tests themselves. By now I was on my sixth pregnancy but I hadn't been treated by St Thomas' at that time. They were still doing the tests.

'I was in London doing a presentation at the Savoy, part of my job as a product manager, and I remember thinking "should I be doing this?" I was seven weeks pregnant. The work went well but the next day I had a miscarriage. When I went to the hospital they scanned me and said they had found another heartbeat, which meant I must have been having twins. I thought, I can't cope with this, it's such a rollercoaster. I was elated by the news and I was so hopeful that this time things would be fine. But then sadly three weeks later when we were on holiday in the Lake District I had to be rushed to hospital and I lost the other twin. I think that was the worst miscarriage, I was very distressed.

'I seriously considered having a hysterectomy so I wouldn't have to keep going through all this, it was taking over our lives. The team at St Thomas' had made me realize that my chances were slimmer than I had thought. They made me face reality that it was highly likely that I wouldn't be able to carry a baby. This sounds odd but I welcomed the news, that level of honesty. In the past I had been told I was just unlucky. They were the first people who understood what I was going through and they talked straight to me so I knew what to expect.

'At St Thomas' I had some more tests. I felt that I couldn't cope with an eighth miscarriage but the doctors there said I should give it one last try. They put me on a different type of heparin, and aspirin, to thin my blood.

When I got pregnant I was monitored very closely both by St Thomas' and by my local team in Cambridgeshire. It was a very difficult pregnancy. I did lose a lot of blood and I was sure I would lose the baby. I can remember at 16 weeks after another scare I decided that I couldn't do this any longer, I almost hoped they wouldn't find a heartbeat so it could be all over. I was numb when they scanned and said everything was fine.

'Jade was delivered by Caesarean. The joy I felt was indescribable. People were worried about me because I was so high with it all. I was up and about really quickly. We were home after two days and I was so excited I couldn't sleep.

'I think if I hadn't pushed to see the right people I wouldn't have my beautiful baby or the happy and stable relationship that David and I have today. I would have given up on starting a family and thrown myself into my job.

'I would say to other women that they should look for the symptoms and don't be one of the herd. Everyone is so individual, each woman has to make sure she is doing the best for herself and her baby. Listen to the doctors but if there are any doubts don't hesitate to get a second opinion. What happened to us is proof that it is worth fighting to get the right treatment.'

Anna Divers

Anna Divers from Faversham in Kent was luckier than most because she was diagnosed with Hughes syndrome after only two miscarriages. But Anna, a systems development manager, says she still found it tough to cope with the loss.

'I first became pregnant in August 1997. My husband Nigel and I were so overjoyed that we told everyone straight away. At eight weeks there was a bit of spotting and I went for an early scan just to make sure everything was all right. Sure enough they found a heartbeat. But one week later the bleeding got heavier and a further scan showed no heartbeat, just an empty sac. I had a kind of D and C ('dilation and curettage' – a gynaecological procedure) to ensure everything was removed to prevent infection and that was it – no advice, no counselling; we were just told this was very common. That didn't help us at all. We were devastated, it had never crossed our minds that such a thing might happen to us. I threw myself into my work as a way of coping, we didn't have the courage to try again until 2000.

'In the July I became pregnant again, this time we told no one; we were scared it might all go wrong again. And it did. I miscarried at nine weeks with exactly the same symptoms, one week spotting but a scan showing all was well, then the next week nothing.

'I was convinced this wasn't just "one of those things". I thought that something might be wrong with the environment the baby was trying to grow in, even though I had lived like a nun this time round. I felt stronger than the first time, I was determined to find out why this had happened, even though I knew that in Britain doctors don't normally investigate two recurrent miscarriages, you normally have to suffer the agony of three. By chance I saw a different doctor and she suggested I go for a blood test. It was found I had the antiphospholipid antibody which I was told caused the blood to become sticky and in pregnancy made the blood flow through the placenta poor, causing problems for the growing baby.'

Anna was referred to a gynaecologist at Kent and Canterbury Hospital who specialized in this field. Anna became pregnant in April 2001 and was put on daily injections of heparin and low-dose aspirin, both to thin the blood.

'I was fortunate enough to attend the foetal medicine unit at the hospital and that gave me tremendous reassurance. The scans started early, at six weeks. When they did the second one at seven weeks I heard one of the team say "How many did we see last week?" which threw me completely. Then I realized there were two heartbeats – we were having twins!

'I'm not religious but it seemed almost as if having twins was somehow making up for the two I had lost before. After that I said a prayer every day of my pregnancy.

'On 12 December Harry and Jack arrived. I was proud that they were delivered normally and that I had gone to 39 weeks. They were excellent weights: 6 lb 13 oz (3.1 kg) and 5 lb 10 oz (2.6 kg). I am certain this was because the blood flow was so good, owing to the treatment I was on.

'I still can't believe the twins are here, I owe so much to Dr Scarlett who was the one who sent me for the simple blood test that made the successful pregnancy possible and gave us Harry and Jack.'

Maria Pepe

'When I first became pregnant I was 36 years old and in good health. I was fit, active and under no particular stress. Everything had gone well up to week 29 of the pregnancy. It was then that I became aware that I hadn't felt the baby move for a day or so. I wasn't particularly worried as he wasn't much of a kicker anyway but we went to the hospital for reassurance. Unfortunately we got a shock, the baby had died.

'The post-mortem that followed showed that the placenta had sheared away from the womb but it wasn't clear why that had happened. Several tests revealed nothing until the results came back from one of my blood tests. It showed I had antiphospholipid antibodies, known as sticky blood. The doctors thought that could have been the reason for a blockage in the placenta which led to the death of my baby.

'The next year I became pregnant again and I was referred to Dr Khamashta at St Thomas'. He recommended aspirin, and an injection of heparin daily to thin my blood. I also had regular ultrasound scans to monitor the blood flow to and from the placenta. The pregnancy went well and three weeks ahead of time our son Tadek was born by Caesarean. He arrived weighing 6 lb 4 oz (2.8 kg) in radiant health. It was wonderful'.

Of all the areas covered in this book this is the one that brings the most hope and good news. For the relatively small cost and effort of screening for and monitoring 'sticky blood' in the early stages of pregnancy so many women and families could be saved the agony of repeated miscarriage.

4

Stroke

Stroke is one of the biggest killers in developed countries: in the USA for example someone suffers a stroke every 53 seconds. It is also one of the most costly conditions as those who survive a stroke can need a lot of medical care. It is the largest single cause of severe disability. The annual cost of treating stroke patients is considerable, estimated at £2.3 billion in the UK and a massive £23 billion in the USA. When people talk of stroke they imagine an older person, probably someone who has had a lifetime of physical neglect. Too much alcohol, too many cigarettes, coupled with stress, a bad diet and no exercise. But the reality is anyone can suffer a stroke, young and old alike. How many times do you hear the story of the man in his mid-30s who doesn't smoke, watches his weight and takes exercise, who then collapses on the squash court with a stroke. It might be an apocryphal tale but it carries a distinct echo of truth with it.

What is a stroke? In simple terms it refers to the sudden onset of symptoms when part of the brain is deprived of blood and oxygen. Although there are some well-known causes of stroke, like high blood pressure, in most cases doctors do not know what triggers it. The medical world has traditionally regarded a stroke to be the result of a haemorrhage – bleeding in the brain. Now ground-breaking research into the effects of Hughes syndrome point to another factor that can cause a stroke – thrombosis or blood clotting: the blood thickens and cuts supply to parts of the brain, starving the area of oxygen and leading to a stroke.

A study in Spain of stroke patients showed that 7 per cent had 'sticky blood'. Further work by a team in Rome looked at so-called 'young strokes' involving people under the age of 45. The results were staggering. It showed that 16 per cent of these patients had the antiphospholipid antibody. The conclusion drawn from this information is that as many as one in five strokes involving people aged 45 and under are due to Hughes syndrome. Dr Hughes and his team regard this as a highly significant discovery. These findings bring fresh hope to victims and potential victims of stroke. Establishing a new identifiable cause of this condition means some cases could be treated more effectively using anticoagulants to thin the blood. It also means that in the cases where people are thought to be at risk of having 'sticky blood', like those who have had a thrombosis or severe headaches, it is possible to prevent a stroke from happening by treating the condition. Even when there is no previous medical history, if a young person has a stroke Dr Hughes believes he or she should be tested as a matter of course. If there is no antibody present then further episodes could, potentially, be prevented or the damage done by the stroke limited.

James Dorrington-Ward

James Dorrington-Ward is a perfect example of how stroke can suddenly appear out of nowhere, even among young and apparently healthy people. When he was 18 James decided to take a gap year and travel across South America with a group of friends. For him it was the trip of a lifetime before getting his head down and working hard at Southampton University. The group had been to Chile and Bolivia, the next stop was to tackle the Inca Trail that would take them to a summit 14 000 ft (4 270 m) above sea level.

They had been at 10 000 ft (3 050 m) for a month before starting on the trail so they all, including James, were well acclimatized. As they made their way higher and higher James became more and more fatigued. He blamed himself for not eating and drinking properly – he put his tiredness down to being terribly unfit. But it wasn't the lack of training that was leaving him gasping for air.

'On the second day we were going up a steep climb, it was hot but there was a cold wind so I couldn't take off any clothes despite the fact that I was sweating badly. I was struggling for breath and felt incredibly tired, I just thought I was out of shape. It got to the point where the others were pushing me up, it was embarrassing. We got to a plateau at lunchtime. I couldn't eat or drink even though I was thirsty, I just wanted to sleep.

'There was only 400 ft (120 m) to go to the top but it was very very steep. The others went on as they could see I was in bad shape, the guide stayed with me. I started walking the last bit, fifty steps at a time. I managed three lots and then I fell to the ground. I was completely disorientated and I remember wondering why I couldn't feel my left side. It was as though that part of my body had just shut down. I felt no pain in my side or in my head, nothing, but there I was on the floor. Once again I just thought it was out of tiredness, I had been suffering from altitude sickness for some time before this climb. I was helped up and recovered enough to sit on a rock. I still couldn't feel my left side. It wasn't frightening because I didn't understand then what was happening. Some of my strength came back and I got angry with myself for letting the others down. I forced myself to get to the top.

'On the way down I had to use a stick as I was limping. We all went down to 13 500 ft (4 115 m) where the camp was. I had about 50 per cent mobility in my left leg. I went to bed and slept. But I woke in the night to find my body shaking violently, I was having the first of many epileptic fits. I couldn't move or speak. The fit lasted about five minutes.'

The next morning the porters had to carry James down the next part of the trail to where there were donkeys that could take him back to the bottom of the mountain. 'At that time I kept having more shakes and I had a huge fit. It was then that I began to feel afraid, I just thought "Oh my God I can't control this".' But James noticed that he began to feel better as soon as he was no longer at high altitude.

Once off the trail he was taken to a small local hospital as an emergency patient and put on a drip. Facilities were limited and he was moved to a larger hospital in Lima where a brain scan was carried out. The suspicions were that James had suffered a stroke but the scan showed nothing. The priority was to get him home to the UK. His parents, who were on holiday in France, were horrified to hear the news. They abandoned their trip and headed home to Dorset to be reunited with their ailing son.

James was seen at Dorchester Hospital where they did a another scan, which revealed lesions or white marks. 'I was told that I had suffered a stroke and had a form of lupus. I was put on high-dose warfarin. But my family and I weren't happy with the diagnosis, we felt it wasn't right. I was lucky that my uncle who is a doctor knew Dr Hughes at St Thomas' and arranged for me to see him. At the time I hadn't heard of 'sticky blood', it certainly wasn't something the doctors at Dorchester knew about'.

Tests showed that James did not have lupus but revealed antiphospholipid antibodies; he had Hughes syndrome. The stickier-than-normal blood and extremely high altitude triggered the stroke and fits. At great heights it becomes more difficult to get oxygen into the blood. James didn't become ill at altitudes on aircraft because the cabin is pressurized. If James had not gone on that trail he might never have learnt that he had this condition.

'I was relieved because I realized that Hughes syndrome wasn't as bad as lupus. I didn't have to have the heparin injections, instead I was prescribed simple aspirin. And it worked.'

Five years later James is still taking aspirin and has had no recurrence of the stroke or fits. He is currently working to qualify as an accountant and says he is so well that he finds it hard to believe what happened to him on that hostile mountainside in Peru.

Dr Hughes says cases like that of James' where there were no previous medical problems are unusual. Although he has seen children as young as four who have suffered a stroke and test positive for 'sticky blood', 'in James' case the assumption was that the tendency to "sticky blood" had been present for some time, but that the conditions at high altitude conspired to produce an actual blood clot.'

More common are those patients who have had a long history of illness and have suffered what are known as 'warning' strokes, or might not even realize they have had a series of strokes until a brain scan has been carried out following other symptoms.

Janine Billet

Janine Billet has had a lifetime of illness. When she was only ten she had severe headaches followed by aching muscles and joints. Doctors dismissed it as growing pains, but the trouble was they didn't go away when she stopped growing, they just got worse.

Now aged 45 her medical history charts years of suffering and uncertainty. Although she has two healthy children who are in their 20s Janine had five miscarriages before she was 26. She had numerous painful DVTs in her arms and legs. She continued to have headaches and had severe internal bleeding that led to an early hysterectomy. To make matters worse for most of her life she did not know what was wrong.

Despite all these set-backs Janine was a fighter, she was determined not to give in to her illness. She had always had an agile brain, she started her working career in Preston as a bookmaker's settler – having to quickly add up figures. As the years went by she began to notice that she was slowing down. 'I found that I got befuddled with figures. I decided to work for myself as a market trader. And then my grasp of words was affected, my daughter would laugh when I would tell her to "Get the umbrella from the drawer" when I meant knife.

'I have always enjoyed doing crosswords in the newspapers. I found the *Daily Mail* so easy that I would rocket through it, solving the clues as quickly as I could write the answers. The *Daily Telegraph* cryptic crossword took a bit more time but it was rare that I hadn't finished it by lunchtime.'

As her condition worsened she found that not only did she have difficulty getting the answers, she could hardly read and understand the clues. Janine knew something was terribly wrong but had no idea what.

Whatever was behind her deteriorating mind Janine would not to be beaten. She decided to become a mature student studying psychology at Lancaster University. In her first year, when she was 33 years old, she had a stroke. 'It was the worst thing that happened to me. It left me weak on one side and permanently damaged my peripheral vision. It robbed me of a lot of my vocabulary. I found it difficult to do the essays because although I knew the words I wanted to use I couldn't get them out. The tutors would come to me and point out that I had written the exact opposite of what I meant. Luckily they were very supportive. I had only done one term and everyone thought that would be it, that I would have to give up my studies. But the university were very good and said that I should take the exam at the end of the first year. No one expected me to get through it, including myself. I was flabbergasted when I passed. That proved to me that I should carry on as normal. I was determined to finish the course. 'It was quite a moment for me when I got the degree with honours, I had succeeded. I am a positive person and I believe that is what helped me reach my goal.'

But ill health dogged Janine as she struggled through university, 'It was exceptionally hard as I was having difficulty breathing, I had serious chest pains. After leaving Lancaster I ended up in a wheelchair unable to do much for myself, my memory was appalling. I forgot how to do basic things like how to switch on a TV or washing machine. I was being admitted to hospital on a regular basis at this point. I had one episode which the doctors believed was a pulmonary embolism. I survived and they said that I must have an angel on my shoulder.

'By early 1997 I was becoming desperate to find out what was wrong with me. I was seeing a number of doctors in different areas of medicine – a neurologist, urologist, ophthalmologist, cardiologist, to name but a few. Each one was treating the symptoms in isolation. It was suggested I had ME or MS. Not one of the doctors looked at the whole picture. It was implied I was a hysterical patient. Out of desperation I agreed to see a psychiatrist. He assured me that my problems were definitely medical, although he was surprised that I wasn't suffering from reactive depression triggered by the lack of support I had received. He referred me to Dr Hughes at St Thomas'. It was the best thing anyone could have done.

'I arrived at the hospital in a wheelchair, I was a very sick woman. To my utter relief Dr Hughes did not rubbish my symptoms, he understood what was wrong and for the first time in years I had some hope. After my first consultation I began to feel there was light at the end of my very dark personal tunnel. Tests were done which showed I had Hughes syndrome. I was treated with anticoagulants and gradually I found it easier to breathe and my memory began to return. After a few months the wheelchair was stored away and I used the stair lift less and less'.

For the first time as an adult Janine felt she had a good quality of life and there was hope for her future. These days she is racing through the crosswords again; if she finds they become difficult she knows it is a sign her condition is flaring and she needs to increase her medication.

Lynda Smock

Lynda Smock had a stroke in May 2001, something that puzzled the doctors in her home town in Arizona, USA. Lynda was 40, didn't smoke or drink, had low blood pressure and was only marginally overweight.

'I had the stroke at home and all the doctors I saw just shrugged their shoulders and said they didn't know why it had happened to me. I was told to take one aspirin a day and I would be fine.

'A few weeks later I had a second, much bigger stroke. That got their attention! I was in the emergency area of the hospital, I lay in my bed praying for God to send the right doctor to me. I refused to tell them the name of my neurologist because I thought he was an idiot. So the team at the hospital brought in a specialist who literally saved my life. He asked if he could test for a special disease that has migraines and miscarriages as symptoms in earlier life with strokes and heart attacks following later on.

'I have two healthy teenagers but I did have three miscarriages when I was younger and I had a history of migraines; I was also hospitalized when I was six with a blood disorder'.

Lynda agreed to have blood tests and they showed she did have 'sticky blood'. She was given anticoagulants and appeared to recover. Five months later she was taken off the medication as she was about to have an operation.

'I had a third stroke, they simply hadn't given me enough heparin to prevent it in the run up to the operation. They increased the dose and the symptoms of the stroke left me with only minimal memory damage and some tiring on the right side.

'My children now live with the worry that Mom might have a stroke and not recover. They call me throughout the day to make sure I am OK. It is a shame as they no longer have the innocence and confidence they should have because their Mom isn't "supermom" anymore, she gets tired and cranky whereas before I was the most patient soul around. My husband is concerned that I won't live to see my grandbabies, I don't expect there'll be any for ten to twelve years but I want to be there for my children to help them celebrate a new generation of life.'

Lynda is convinced Hughes syndrome runs in her family. Once she got a diagnosis she began to retrace her relative's medical history and she feels certain it has been responsible for deaths in three generations of her family.

'My grandfather William was bedridden for the last two years of his life with horrid headaches and partial paralysis on one side. His death certificate says brain tumour but we wonder if it wasn't antiphospholipid syndrome; this all happened back in 1939 in Kentucky so there is no way we could ever be sure. My Mom died of an apparent heart attack at 55. We have no history in the family of heart disease, Mom had been to hospital twice with headaches, chest pains and feeling very tired. Tests on her heart showed it was fine; looking back I think a blood clot was the culprit as the coroner said the heart had been starved of oxygen.

'Then my brother Michael died in his sleep, when he was 44. It was a stroke. No one could understand why, perhaps that was a "sticky blood" clot.'

Lynda plans to see if Hughes syndrome has affected the next generation of her family; she and her husband will have tests done on their children in the future to see if they have the antibody.

'Without a strong faith in God and a family to laugh and help me through the tough times I think I would have gone mad and given up. These days I am constantly cautious about what I eat and do, in the face of this disease my life has changed forever.'

5

Headaches

When you talk to patients with Hughes syndrome it is striking that the single most common symptom they suffer from is a recurrent severe headache. We all have headaches from time to time but in people with 'sticky blood' it can be a warning sign that something else is wrong. If you imagine the fine capillaries in the brain becoming clogged or the blood flow being restricted because it is too sticky then you can see why it might cause pain in the head. Because headache isn't usually something to make you rush to the doctor's surgery, most people take a few painkillers and forget about it. In those with Hughes syndrome, however, headache could be the first indicator that the disease is present. Many patients say they began to have headaches when they were teenagers, and that the pain became an untreated feature of their lives. It was only later they developed other aspects of 'sticky blood'. There is also evidence that women can have the 'sticky blood' headache during or after pregnancy when their blood will be thicker because of their condition.

In a large number of cases that arrive at the clinic in St Thomas' the headaches come with other symptoms, such as flashing lights, nausea and vomiting. Migraine sufferers will recognize the unpleasant features of this kind of attack. At present there is no cure for true migraine, as it's known, although there is an array of drugs to relieve the symptoms. If it transpired that Hughes syndrome triggered migraine, then it would certainly be possible to treat and prevent it.

Dr Hughes predicts that 'sticky blood' will become an important, recognized cause of migraine, even more important than the link between this condition and the adverse reactions caused by taking the contraceptive pill. But it will take time to put those pieces of the jigsaw together; as Hughes syndrome is still a relatively new disease there is little research into this link. The Rayne Institute at St Thomas' has done a trial with some patients to see if anticoagulation helps Hughes syndrome patients who have debilitating headaches. The results are impressive; people with intractable migraine say the pain disappears once the drugs are started.

Such findings could have broad implications for the treatment of headache, and of migraine in particular. It will be necessary though to push for more research to examine these early findings. The best witnesses to this 'miracle' cure are the patients themselves.

Jaine Foster

Jaine Foster had never suffered badly from headaches until her second pregnancy. She did have a history of illness though. Diagnosed as having rheumatoid arthritis when she was 16, she developed deformities of some joints and needed corrective surgery. It was when she was 21 that tests showed she was actually suffering from lupus; the drugs she'd been given all those years for the arthritis were ineffective. This meant the lupus had been untreated and thereby allowed to do damage which Jaine now feels could have been avoided if she had been given an earlier diagnosis; but twenty-two years ago doctors didn't look for lupus, never mind Hughes syndrome. Like many sufferers of lupus and 'sticky blood' she had problems getting pregnant; she and her husband decided to try IVF (in-vitro fertilization).

It worked and they had a baby daughter, Jasmine. Four years later the couple tried for their second child. It was while she was pregnant with Oliver that Jaine experienced the worst, most gruelling pain she has ever known.

'At fifteen weeks I started to get a very bad headache. It was an intense pain but worst of all was nothing seemed to stop it. I tried the lot, I went to the chemist and asked for everything and anything to stop my head hurting. It felt as though I had a skull cap on that was far too tight. The pain was there when I went to sleep and when I woke up. I became desperate, I just kept thinking that it would never go away, that I would always feel this bad. I tried relaxation tapes, reflexology, headache pills, migraine pills, stress relief pills; but it was no good, the nightmare just went on.

'As I got nearer to the due date I comforted myself with the thought that the pregnancy was the cause of the headache and that once I had given birth it would go away and let me get on with my life.

'I had Oliver and sure enough it did go. I was delighted.'

Her joy was to be short-lived. Two weeks later the headache returned with a vengeance. The pain was so severe that it robbed Jaine of her ability to enjoy her new baby. It put her under enormous pressure as she had the baby and Jasmine to care for.

Her husband Richard did what he could but Jaine became depressed at the seemingly incurable pain in her head.

'I cried a lot at that time. I had this baby that wouldn't sleep and a head that wouldn't stop hurting, it was pounding and pounding. I was feeding Oliver every two hours and I just thought my whole world was coming to an end. I thought "I am supposed to enjoy this baby that cost a fortune because of the IVF and instead my world is crumbling."

'It felt as though everything was falling apart around me. I got to the point where I knew I couldn't cope. My husband Richard would come home from work and he would take over and let me go to bed. But even then as I went to sleep I knew the pain would be there when I woke. It was dreadful.

'I thought I should be over the moon, instead I couldn't cope any more. I often called the team at the lupus clinic at St Thomas' for support and they were brilliant but it didn't take away the pain. I just wanted to curl up and die.'

The headache was not like a migraine, Jaine says her eyes were not affected. The pain was all over her head, like a bonnet. The painkillers and other treatments made no difference. Richard decided that a weekend away by the seaside might help, Jaine was reluctant to go because she felt so unwell.

Before the trip she went to see Dr Hughes.

Jaine had been tested a number of times for the antiphospholipid antibody. One test was positive, the other two were negative. So she wasn't sure whether or not she had Hughes syndrome, but Dr Hughes decided to put her on a course of heparin injections.

The family went on their trip and Jaine began the medication. 'I remember looking at Richard as I injected myself and saying "look, yet another needle", because I had had so many injections for the IVF.' Jaine had no idea if the heparin would work but she was desperate enough to try anything. She says at one point she literally banged her head hard against a wall just to see if it relieved the pain, needless to say it didn't.

'I woke the next day with this terrible feeling that something was missing. I panicked and went to check on the kids. They were fine, so I started pacing around the room trying to remember what it was that I had misplaced.

'Then it dawned on me. I no longer had the headache. It was completely gone! It was brilliant, the sense of relief is hard to describe. It was sheer joy not to have that grinding pain in my head any more. I felt that at last I could get on with my life.'

Jaine says it took a few more days for the heparin to remove the headache completely. When the course of heparin finished the pain came back so she had to continue with anticoagulant medication. In the two years that have followed, Jaine has been mostly 'headache-free'. She was put on warfarin, which is taken orally so she wouldn't have to inject herself any more. Now she keeps a close watch on her INR. If it becomes too low then she knows the headache will return. These days she knows there is an end to the pain as there are drugs that can help, which means she doesn't have to resort to hitting her head against a brick wall.

Jason Abosch

Hearing about this book, Jason got in touch with me via the internet; he said he wanted to share his story. It helps to know you are not alone; isolation and illness are tough to live with. Sometimes just telling others what you have been through helps you cope with the daily up and downs of a condition such as Hughes syndrome.

Twenty-five-year-old Jason was in excellent health. He worked-out six times a week at his local gym in Baltimore, studying karate. Then in November 2000 his world collapsed.

'I initially woke up with a terrible headache in the morning. Prior to that, I never got headaches. It gradually got worse during the day and by noon, I noticed my vision was beginning to go. My vision continued to deteriorate, the headache persisted and then all of the sudden I had numbness. The numbness began in my arm, proceeded to my leg, and then made its way up to my cheeks, chin and tongue. I also began losing the use of my right hand, was speaking slowly and in a confused manner and suffered some short-term memory loss. From an emotional point of view, I was definitely scared. Until then, I was in excellent physical health. I knew something was not right. I called my physician and visited him later that day.'

Unlike the vast majority of patients in this book, Jason was fortunate to get a diagnosis very quickly. Although his doctor was in the dark about Hughes syndrome, Jason saw a neurologist who was familiar with the condition and recognized the symptoms.

'It took two weeks to diagnose. I went through body scans and brain scans. They gave me a spinal tap (to check the fluid in the spine) and did a lot of blood tests. The blood work revealed the condition. It was somewhat difficult for my physicians to diagnose – this was a rather unknown condition to them. Fortunately, I visited a neurologist who is well read and he knew enough of the condition to test me for it. He, in all likelihood, saved my life. All other tests, other than the blood test, were normal. My symptoms could have easily been dismissed as a freak occurrence.'

Jason was admitted to hospital and found it difficult to deal with the sudden change from being a fighting fit young man to taking a cocktail of medication and being stalked by a fickle and unpredictable illness.

'Having this condition has changed my life. After diagnosis, I spent five days in the stroke unit at a hospital. For a 24-year-old, that is emotionally tough. It is a condition I wrestle with rather routinely. My diet has changed dramatically and I have to be cautious in my daily activities. I get headaches all the time, and stress has a greater effect on me.

'I have spent a total of 15 days or so in the hospital in the last 13 months, I take a handful of pills each day, plus it puts stress on my girlfriend and other family members. There are a lot of little things that one must change, and in the aggregate, they have a profound effect on everyday life.

'My blood is tested every two weeks. I take five medications, including an anticoagulant, an antihypersensitive drug and low-dose aspirin. I visit a specialist at Johns Hopkins Hospital every six months and consult with a neurologist and physician when I need to. I did visit with a psychiatrist for a few months after diagnosis.'

For Jason the diagnosis of 'sticky blood' was devastating and he is struggling to cope with being unwell.

'Things are still much like a roller-coaster. I have reminders of the condition each and every day – sometimes it's headaches, or not being able to eat something or do something, or just taking medication. The thickness of my blood fluctuates a lot, so the levels of my medications often change. The biggest day-to-day problem is headaches and occasionally blurred vision. All of that being said, I consider myself lucky and fortunate. This condition is more of an inconvenience than anything else. There are other medical issues that are ten times worse.'

6

Do You Really Have MS?

One of the most alarming aspects of Hughes syndrome is how easily it can be mistaken for other conditions. As more cases come to light it is clear that Hughes syndrome is often overlooked. This isn't a criticism of doctors who don't spot it, just a reflection of the current lack of awareness about 'sticky blood' – if you are not looking for it the chances are you won't find it.

Perhaps the most dramatic example of this is in relation to multiple sclerosis (MS). No one knows yet how often Hughes syndrome is mistaken for MS. It is still early days and little research has been undertaken to date, but the indications are that a closer look at this cross-over will reveal the numbers are significant. In one recent clinic Dr Hughes saw three patients who had been told they had MS but blood tests showed they were actually suffering from Hughes syndrome. There were about 40 patients at that clinic; a quick bit of mental arithmetic shows just under 10 per cent had mistakenly been told they had MS. Obviously that figure is a rough guide and could be irrelevant beyond the patients who found their way to this particular clinic, which specializes in autoimmune disease, in particular lupus. But there is a growing body of evidence to support the premise that the numbers of people mis-diagnosed could be large – thereby the pressure for greater knowledge is also increasing.

The difference for the patient could not be more profound. Both diseases are incurable and potentially life-threatening. But there are a number of crucial differences. Multiple sclerosis is a progressive degenerative illness. It eats away at the nervous system. A patient faces the prospect of losing his mobility, being confined to a wheelchair, having slurred speech, muscle weakness, double vision and generalized numbness, all of which can get worse throughout his life. The damage done is often permanent. There is no fully acknowledged treatment for MS, although beta-interferon is believed to slow the progress of the disease. The best weapon a patient has is knowledge and courage.

On the flip side, being told you have Hughes syndrome is not good news but in most cases the outlook is nowhere near as tough. Once you get over the shock, and in most cases go away and try to discover what on earth this condition is, then the general picture is more promising. Most important to remember is that the condition is extremely treatable. There are a number of highly effective, inexpensive drugs readily available through the NHS on prescription. And in some cases a prescription isn't required as 'sticky blood' can be controlled with as little as low-dose aspirin. The damage caused is usually not permanent and with the right monitoring the sufferer can expect to lead a relatively normal life.

Over the years doctors in this field have shared a growing concern about how common this mis-diagnosis might be. So the team at St Thomas' decided to analyse a sample of patients on their books. Their research paper was published in 2000 and the result was enough to raise even the most cynical eyebrow.

The research group at the hospital's Rayne Institute, led by Dr Maria Cuadrado, looked at the cases of 27 women patients who had been originally diagnosed as having or highly likely to have MS. They had all attended the clinic over a period of two years. The primary reason for the initial diagnosis was the result of MRI (magnetic resonance imaging) scans of the brain which showed lesions – in lay terms ominous white blobs on the scan that looks like an X-ray of the brain. The lesions are one of the major abnormalities doctors look for when they suspect MS. But for all these patients the devastating news that they had, or most likely had, this appalling disease was not the end of the story. In each case there were symptoms that did not fit the MS picture. And every one of the patients had tested positive for antiphospholipid antibodies. Hence the referral to see Dr Hughes.

As the patients' files were reviewed the facts began to fit together like a jigsaw. A number of the women had suffered miscarriage, some had severe migraines, others suffered from arthritis. The majority also had the white lesions, but that did not necessarily mean they had MS. Most important of all though was the positive blood test for antiphospholipid antibodies.

Staggering as it might sound it transpired that not one of these women had MS, they all were suffering from 'sticky blood'. The group was not a quirk. Since this report was published there have been an increasing number of patients with similar stories to tell. The upshot is Dr Hughes believes blood tests for Hughes syndrome should be carried out in all cases where the diagnosis of MS is unclear.

Jeremiah Johnston-Sheehan

Jeremiah is a talented architect. Now in his early 40s he has always taken care of his health, watching his diet and taking regular exercise. One of his favourite pastimes is hill-walking. So the onset of an incurable illness was particularly hard on him. It was while walking in the Highlands of Scotland that he first noticed the change in his health. He would suddenly feel utterly exhausted, a paralysing fatigue that made it hard for him to even get back to his car. He knew something was wrong and thought it might be linked to the asthma he had suffered from for many years.

Gradually other symptoms developed. 'I started having double vision, the beginnings of optic neuritis. Then I began to trip and had problems with my balance. I had something called drop foot where I couldn't lift my toes so I would fall over them. I was getting badly bruised, at one point I ended up in casualty with dislocated ribs and gashes, I looked as though I had been in a war. The doctors described me as "a medical chaosity".'

He was given an MRI scan. When the results came through his neurologist asked him if he wanted the 'good news' or the 'bad news'. Jeremiah's heart sank, but he went along with the game no matter how inappropriate. He wanted to hear the good first. Relief came with the news that he did not have a brain tumour. But that optimistic moment was immediately crushed by the bad news. There were white markers on the scan. The diagnosis was probable secondary progressive MS.

'At one point I was admitted to St Thomas'. On the ward I was surrounded by people with end-stage MS. I was sitting there looking around wondering if I shared their fate, the condition these people were in was not something you see on TV shows or anywhere else. There I was, at 42, seeing what might be around the corner for me. All I wanted to do was get on with my work but it wasn't going to be that simple.'

Out of all the tests carried out there was one blood result that didn't fit. Jeremiah had antiphospholipid antibodies. 'My neurologist didn't think it was significant but he still felt the proper thing was to check it out by referring me to another specialist.

'I had never heard of Hughes syndrome, so when I got home I hit the internet and within four hours I knew enough to understand that having this and not MS would definitely be "good" news. The trouble was they couldn't do a repeat blood test for months. It was Christmas and my appointment wasn't until the following summer. I forced the neurologist to give me some odds, "sticky blood" v. MS. He said 85 per cent MS and 15 per cent something else. At that point I was resigned to the fact that the only way for me to survive was to carry on as if it was MS. If I was wrong, well so much the better, if not I would have done what I could.'

Jeremiah knew that beta-interferon was the only drug that seemed to slow down the progress of the disease, and the earlier treatment began the better. The drawback was that the NHS would not pay for it. So he and his wife decided to fund the treatment themselves. It cost £700 a month, a lot of money if Jeremiah were to live for the next 30 years or more.

'I had been through two years of feeling very unwell, months of tests and then dealing with the news that I most likely had MS. I elected to start on the beta-interferon partly for the benefit of my wife and family. I felt I had to show them that I was doing something.'

Jeremiah had been referred to consultant rheumatologist and specialist in autoimmune diseases, Dr David D'Cruz, at St Thomas' Hospital. Blood tests were run again to see if the antibody was still present. Jeremiah had to wait for the results; he says it was the longest two weeks of his life.

'When Dr D'Cruz called me back and started to say "In my opinion you do not have MS, you have something called antiphospholipid syndrome . . ." I was overjoyed. I had read so much about 'sticky blood' that I knew exactly what he was saying, it was such incredibly good news and a tremendous relief.'

Once treatment with warfarin began, Jeremiah's symptoms started to disappear. 'The medication kicked in very quickly. The tingling feeling in my fingers and toes went away, as did the double vision. In a matter of days I no longer needed the walking stick and the fatigue started to lift.'

The key to controlling the symptoms is to maintain a delicate balance, to keep an eye on how thin the blood is. Jeremiah does this by using a self-test kit which he bought for £300 and uses at home. It measures the blood's INR, international normalized ratio, which means comparing the thickness of the patient's blood with what you would expect to find in normal blood. Jeremiah feels well when his measurement is 3–4; the higher the ratio the thinner the blood.

'If I have been under great stress, for instance I was made redundant at the end of 2001, then my condition begins to deteriorate. My INR drops and with that the tingling, fatigue, mobility problems, and so on, start to return. I test myself and see that I need to increase the warfarin. And so far this works for me.

'Having had to live with the fear that I had MS was very traumatic, and because of that I do find it harder these days to cope with stress. But I also think that I had a chance to start over again, thanks to the team at St Thomas' where they are inquisitive and challenge things – they ask questions and get answers, which is good news for people like me.'

Dr Sally Evans

Among non-medical people the general consensus is that doctors look after their own. If one of their fraternity becomes ill they are fast-tracked through the NHS minefield and get first-class treatment. The case of Dr Sally Evans shows that is not always true.

Despite her status as GP it took Sally seven years to get the right diagnosis. In that time she suffered some terrible symptoms which did permanent damage to her nervous system. At the age of 40 she has to come to terms with the fact that part of her face will always be numb, she is virtually blind in her right eye, has some problems with her left eye, and is incontinent. In the year 2000 she had to give up her job in a busy local practice in Woking.

'I felt very unhappy for those seven years. I was constantly worrying what was wrong with me, I found it desperately frustrating not having a diagnosis. I began to think I was going mad, I started to think I might be imagining my vertigo, the optic neuritis or that I couldn't feel anything on my face. I had so many costly investigations done, and they showed nothing.'

Sally was seeing two neurologists, she had pushed for a second opinion. She had been told she had multiple sclerosis. 'I will never forget that moment. The consultant shook my hand, told me I had MS and simply said goodbye. And that was it, there was nothing he could do so I was shown the door.'

Fortunately Sally's other neurologist was not convinced. Her brain scan showed no lesions and he felt her symptoms did not follow the pattern of MS. Also Sally's blood test for antiphospho- lipid antibodies was very very high.

Sally had not heard of Hughes syndrome, nor had any of her medical contemporaries. Luckily her neurologist did know the syndrome and so she was referred to Dr Hughes. Tests confirmed that she was suffering from 'sticky blood' and not MS. She was put on warfarin and began to monitor her own INR. But a lot of damage had already been done; perhaps hardest of all is the loss of sight in one eye.

'I will never be able to practise medicine in the future. I did persevere for a few years but it just became too difficult. Imagine working in a GPs' surgery when you are incontinent, or when you cannot see properly. Most of the nerve damage will never improve. The numbness in my face is like having permanent dental injections. When I eat I dribble on one side, my smile is crooked and when I talk to someone I feel as though half my face is frozen. It makes me feel impersonal and detached.

'I am not bitter or angry that it took seven years to get a diagnosis. I know it might seem odd that as a doctor it took so long but then perhaps it was because of my profession that I was more likely to ignore my symptoms. I dismissed things and told myself I was being a bit of a hypochondriac. I was less outspoken about what was going on, and so therefore I am partly responsible.

'One thing I do feel strongly about after being wrongly told I had MS is that doctors should not tell somebody what their diagnosis is until they are absolutely sure. To be told you have a degenerative disease and then that you don't, but have something else unpleasant is a terrible psychological shock.'

7

The Brain

Few things can be more frightening then finding you are losing your memory, speech and vision. To open your mouth and splutter out the wrong words, or struggle to remember events that happened moments before are devastating symptoms. People with early Alzheimer's disease experience this deterioration but it is also a sign that the antiphospholipid antibodies might be present. If that is the case then the news is good, it means that rather than slipping into degenerative Alzheimer's for which there is no cure, you have sticky blood and can be treated, often with highly effective results.

Dr Hughes has found a considerable number of patients come to him complaining of having a 'foggy head'. They recount how their self esteem is damaged because people, work colleagues or friends, who are used to them being on the ball, notice a change and tease them about being slow or dim-witted. The result of treatment is dramatic, patients talk of the fog lifting and seeing things clearly again; they speak of the enormous relief at getting their speech and memory back.

Dr Hughes believes this aspect of the syndrome must be examined more closely: 'Research to date is limited but I feel certain that in time this syndrome will become widely recognized by psychologists and psychiatrists for patients with a variety of neurological disorders.'

Hughes syndrome can also cause major neurological disturbances. Dr Hughes likes to explain the impact of 'sticky blood' on the brain by making an analogy with a car. When the mixture of fuel is too rich the engine begins to stutter and stop working properly. One patient described it to me as being like a computer that has a virus and begins to do odd things out of the user's control.

Clots that appear as white blobs on a brain scan impair the normal function of the brain. Sufferers can have mini-strokes known as TIAs (transient ischaemic attacks). If it is a minor one then the symptoms will be negligible, the patient might not even notice anything wrong. It is a different story if he or she suffers a series of strokes – they can cause permanent damage to the brain affecting areas like memory, speech and vision.

Barbara Osborn

Barbara Osborn thought she was going to die. In a matter of weeks the former British Airways stewardess was transformed from a healthy, energetic mother of two into someone who was unable to walk and in constant need of help from others. Barbara was consigned to a wheelchair, attacked by muscle spasms that were so violent she lost control of her body. Devastated by the mystery illness she contemplated suicide. Barbara, who was 38 at the time, had been preparing to go back to work as her children were eleven and six. 'The first thing I noticed was that my legs felt heavy when I was running up stairs – I was the kind of person who was always rushing everywhere. The heaviness would come and go and I didn't think much of it. But then it became more frequent and I thought I had better see my doctor,' says Barbara, who lives in Reigate with her husband, Robert, the managing director of a construction company.

She was referred to a neurologist but in the following months her condition deteriorated. Her legs would suddenly give way under her and she found it difficult to get out of bed without help. Worst of all she didn't know what was wrong as there was no diagnosis. Barbara and her doctors thought she had multiple sclerosis. 'They took me in for tests and I spent ten days on a ward with people who had MS, some of whom were in the final stages of the disease. It was very grim and I was so frightened, watching these people dying and thinking that I would soon be just as sick as they were. I had got it into my head this was what I had. And although the tests didn't confirm I had MS, the doctors said it was still possible I did have it.'

Barbara's condition worsened. She became so unwell and unable to control her body that she could no longer walk. 'The spasms were like having an electric current shooting through my body lifting my feet off the ground. On one occasion a spasm was so strong that it threw me backwards onto the coffee table splitting my head open and I had to be rushed to hospital.

'At one point I felt terribly low, because I believed I was becoming such a burden on my husband and children. It was then that I understood why people committed suicide. I thought in a cold logical way about it as the only thing I could do to relieve the suffering I had brought on my family.' But Barbara struggled on against the illness. The frustrating thing was that despite endless tests, she still didn't know what was wrong.

Then there was a breakthrough. Something abnormal showed up in a blood test and Barbara was referred to a rheumatologist. She was told that it was thought she had lupus.

'I had never heard of lupus and the doctor was so vague in explaining it that I thought I must have that disease *and* MS. My friends went to local libraries and read about it. The books were pretty old and painted a bleak picture. They all thought I was on my way out. There was so little information available about lupus, even six years ago.

'One of my friends found the name of the leading specialist in this field, Dr Hughes at St Thomas' in London. So I insisted I saw him. One of the first things he said to me was "I bet they've told you that you have MS, well, we will see about that".'

Dr Hughes says Barbara's case was the worst he had seen. He was certain that she did not have MS: 'Barbara was suffering from lupus but I also felt that she had the classic symptoms of Hughes syndrome.'

After months of suffering, an inexpensive blood test was all that was needed to confirm that Barbara did not have MS but had Hughes syndrome as well as lupus. Once she was treated with a drug that thins the blood her recovery was staggering. Within 48 hours the spasms had gone.

'The change was so dramatic after I started taking warfarin. I found the spasms had stopped and things started to improve within days, I could hardly believe it. I could get myself out of bed and I was out of the wheelchair pretty quickly, then I walked with the help of sticks for about six months.'

The wheelchair and sticks have long gone. Barbara shows little outward sign of the trauma she went through. Tall and slim, she walks unaided and is every bit as energetic as she was when the illness struck six years ago. Barbara is still on medication and has her own blood test machine to monitor her INR levels. She says she can tell when she is becoming ill again because her speech becomes muddled.

Barbara has dedicated her time to working for the charity that helps fund the lupus unit at St Thomas' Hospital in central London – the largest of its kind in the world with 2 500 patients registered. Barbara is also a key figure in the Hughes Syndrome

Foundation, the charity set up to improve awareness of this condition.

Jon Barber

When I rang Jon Barber he cheerfully told me the moment he put down the phone he wouldn't remember one word of our conversation. The damage to his brain by repeated TIAs and strokes means he has virtually no short-term memory. 'I don't have any friends these days because I can't remember anyone. I know those who have made it to the long-term part of my memory but all the rest is a blank.' Jon, a former engineer, puts a brave and jovial veneer on how badly Hughes syndrome has affected him and those around him.

It was while doing the school run that his life changed forever. 'I was 41 when it all began to happen. I was driving my 11-year-old daughter to school. During the journey we had a heated argument about her not doing homework and missing school. I was driving back home when I got this incredible pain in my chest and I thought: "Here we go, I am having a heart attack." I went to hospital and had a second episode while they were examining me. They did a number of tests but could find no damage to my heart but said that I had suffered two massive angina attacks. They sent me up to St Thomas' to have more tests. The results were clear and the specialist said he wished his heart would be as strong as mine when he got to my age, he said I had the heart of a 16-year-old.'

'A few months later I had another violent episode. Once again they found nothing, they told me none of the right enzymes were present in the blood to show there had been a heart attack. I saw a cardiologist near our home in Worthing and he said he could find nothing wrong with me. I was given a range of tablets and that was it.'

But Jon did not recover, his condition worsened. He was frustrated and depressed by the lack of a diagnosis. Jon's work suffered and he lost his job. He had a few more painful attacks and then started to lose his speech. 'I found early on there were certain words missing. One of the first to go was the word "chess". I was talking to my daughter who was trying to describe the game to me and I had no idea what she meant, I simply couldn't grasp what the word meant. I lost that particular word for a couple of months then it came back suddenly when we were watching a game show and the question was "what is the game that uses knights and castles" and I blurted out "chess".

'Then in August 1999, on the night of the lunar eclipse I got a blind spot in my left eye. There was this huge white blob in my vision and an indescribable pain in the back of my head. I had a tooth out once without an anaesthetic and the pain beats that, it would be pleasant in comparison. The next day I went to the optician and he said I should go to hospital straight away as the damage he could see was consistent with a stroke. Instead I made an appointment to see my doctor the following day. I went home to have a cup of tea and a think about what was happening to me. It was then I had another blind spot.'

Jon was due to see the chief ophthalmologist at his local hospital when he had a massive stroke. He lost his voice and the sight in his left eye. 'It happened while I was in bed, I had just woken up and I was almost blind and I couldn't speak. They did lots of tests, I had ultrasounds, CT (computed tomographic) and MRI scans.'

The tests confirmed Jon had suffered a major stroke, there was also evidence of hundreds of mini-strokes; one area of the brain on his scan showed substantial damage. 'I am told I had between 250 and 350 mini-strokes. On the scans you can see a chunk of my brain is missing on the frontal right side, the part that deals with memory.

'Three weeks after I got home from hospital I was still virtually blind and had no voice. My ophthalmologist said there was no way the sight in my left eye would come back, there was also doubt my voice would return.

'I am a Christian, every year I go down to a special gathering in Minehead called Spring Harvest, I work as a steward. I feared this year I would not make it. Then I woke up at 4 am one morning and I had this sure knowledge I would get my sight and my voice back. I knew I would ride my motorbike, a Honda GL700, down to Minehead and be a steward. It was my dearest wish.

'Each day after that there was an improvement in both my speech and sight. Oddly, and embarrassingly, the first words that came back to me were some Arabic swearwords I learnt while I was in the army.

'Within two weeks I was well on the road to recovery. My neurologist said he had never seen anything like it, he was shocked by how quickly I got my voice back. And that certainty in the early hours of the morning was right, I was able to go to the Spring Harvest festival in Minehead on my motorbike and I was well enough to be a steward.'

But there was no miracle cure for Jon's overall condition which still didn't have a name. He had been ill for some years and was desperate to know what was going on. He saw a neurologist who told Jon he might have 'sticky blood'. Jon immediately went on the internet to find out what it was. He discovered he wasn't alone in suffering this terrible autoimmune disease. He linked up with other people who had the same symptoms and agonizing journey to diagnosis. It was on the net he came across the name Dr Graham Hughes at St Thomas' in London. Jon saw his GP and insisted on a referral.

'Dr Hughes took one look at me and said I had classic symptoms of Hughes syndrome. He put me on warfarin and it is marvellous how well it works.'

Within weeks things had improved dramatically.

'I used to have TIAs all the time. I have only had two since I started taking the warfarin in September 2001. Under normal circumstances I would have had a hundred of them by now. Bits of memory have come back but other bits are lost for ever. I find I sometimes think I know something but when I search my brain for it there is nothing but a black hole.

'These days I feel much more confident that I can go out and something won't happen to me, at one point I was housebound for fear of having a TIA on the street. My wife and two children have more freedom because I don't need a minder when I leave the house. I still suffer from depression and a few other symptoms but in general I have got my quality of life back.

'How would I describe "sticky blood"? It is like driving along a motorway in a thick fog, you can't see properly no matter how you try, when you take the warfarin the fog lifts and suddenly you can see clearly again. It is a blessed relief.'

8

The Heart

One of the most dangerous aspects of Hughes syndrome is the fact clots can develop in the arteries, giving the disease access to the major organs where serious damage can be done. The heart is then vulnerable and patients might have a coronary thrombosis, or heart attack. They can also suffer painful angina attacks. Frustratingly for them it is often the case that the usual tests for angina or coronary problems come up negative, giving the individual a clean bill of health when everyone, doctors included, knows that the person has suffered a serious episode of some kind. Current evidence shows that the involvement of 'sticky blood' in coronary problems is less common than in other areas, like clots in the brain or miscarriage.

Nevertheless, it is still a field cardiologists should look at closely. It might be the case that knowing someone has the antiphospholipid antibodies would help in their treatment during or after a heart attack. For instance, a different type of anticoagulant drug might provide better results for people in this category or a more aggressive approach to treatment might be required. For some, the heart attack comes after years of struggling to find out what is wrong with their body, why the myriad of symptoms don't add up and leave GPs shaking their heads mystified by the long list of symptoms.

Kay Thackray

Kay Thackray had a heart attack when she was 37 years old. The coronary thrombosis was not the beginning of her story, more the climax. Kay had suffered migraine since she was 14. As she got older the feeling was she probably suffered from MS because of her blurred and double vision, pins-and-needles, fatigue and muscle pain. At one point she was diagnosed as having an overactive thyroid. As she was being treated for this her general health deteriorated.

'The most awful thing was my worsening eyesight, it was so irritating. I could no longer read comfortably and the computer at work would reduce me to tears of frustration. I couldn't read as the words jumped all over the page and I couldn't hold a newspaper out to read it as my arms were like lead weights and ached continually.'

Kay's memory started to fail, she would forget what she was talking about in the midst of a conversation. 'My memory became so poor it was like my mind was a thick fog and I had to wade through it to recall things. I would do something and five minutes later I had no recollection of it at all.

'I kept a diary of my daily symptoms; by now they were so weird I was trying to convince myself they were real. One night my fingers on one hand went numb one by one and then gradually came back one by one. Another time my co-ordination was so poor I couldn't undo some buttons on a child's shirt at the local swimming pool. I would show the diary to my GP, he would read it and shake his head in puzzlement.'

The day Kay had her heart attack she had been busy chasing around doing chores in the morning, it was when she was on her way home the pain began. 'As I drove home I felt a pain in my chest like indigestion. It very quickly got a lot worse and I knew I was having a heart attack. I felt strangely calm and drove to the local surgery. I parked the car, said good morning to an acquaintance on my way in. Once safe inside the surgery I sank to the floor in complete agony.'

Kay's GP thought she was an unlikely candidate for a heart attack but the electrocardiogram (ECG) confirmed her fears. An ambulance came to take her to hospital as an emergency patient. She was given a 'clot buster' and monitored closely for 24 hours in the cardiac unit.

'They did ask me if I wanted a clot buster but my head was spinning with the painkiller I had been given. The doctor told me I needed it because I almost certainly had suffered a heart attack but I remember him warning me that once I had been given it I could bleed from absolutely anywhere in my body and they might not be able to stop it. For the first time I was terrified but I agreed to have it.

'As I lay there in bed with this drug dripping into me I imagined I would bleed to death at any moment but strangely my overall feeling was still one of calm. The whole experience was surreal, as though I was watching all this happen to someone else. The medical team say I was smiling the whole time. Perhaps it was the diamorphine.

'Once I was on the ward I had twice daily heparin injections and aspirin. On the second day a lady came around with library books. I explained I couldn't see well enough to read but she insisted I try one with large print. To get rid of her I gave in and took one. To my amazement I could read, my eyes were totally clear! It was a miracle and I read constantly after that for the sheer joy of it. I felt ecstatic and puzzled as to why this had happened but whatever the reason I didn't care, the main thing was I could read again.'

Kay recovered and was discharged. She felt better than she had for a year or more as most of her symptoms had disappeared although it was a mystery why. Later that year, though, she suffered a full-blown angina attack. An angiogram, which shows whether arteries are blocked, was carried out and Kay got the all clear. 'I had completely clear arteries around my heart. They told me they were wide enough to drive a double-decker bus down.'

At this point one of the tests was for anticardiolipin antibodies; the result was positive. Kay says she wasn't told at the time and it was only later while seeing a haematologist that she saw him write down the words 'lupus anticoagulant'. She had never heard of it but what this meant was at last she had a name for the illness that was causing her symptoms.

Kay went on the internet and discovered there were plenty of others out there like her. She read everything she could about the condition and realized she should be on warfarin, she felt certain she had Hughes syndrome. During her research she came across details of Dr Hughes and begged her GP to give her a referral. While she was waiting for her appointment Kay ended up in hospital again with unstable angina. This time though things were different. She was treated by a young doctor who knew about 'sticky blood'. 'He couldn't understand why I wasn't on warfarin. He said I had tested positive for the antibodies and if a heart attack wasn't a major clotting incident what was? I could have hugged him, I was slowly discovering that doctors who understand Hughes syndrome are like gold dust, a rare breed to be treasured.'

Kay and her husband travelled from Sleaford in Lincolnshire to see Dr Hughes. His diagnosis was exactly what she had expected. 'Dr Hughes said I had described the symptoms of antiphospholipid syndrome and the best thing for me was to be on warfarin. He said if I had been taking it ten years ago I would never have had a heart attack. And without warfarin the risk of another blood clot in the next ten years was 50:50.

'Dr Hughes advised me the warfarin treatment should be lifelong, if I did this I would be "home and dry". Those words were so uplifting and I often tell myself when life seems difficult that I am "home and dry", it never fails to cheer me up.'

9

Lupus and 'Sticky Blood'

It was while he was working with lupus patients in the 1970s that Dr Hughes first noticed the tendency of blood to clot too quickly in some of his patients. That observation led to clinical tests and the discovery that antiphospholipid antibodies (aPL) were present in a large number of patients and were strongly linked to thrombosis in lupus. In some areas the link was so strong it was felt that the presence of these antibodies warranted recognition as a sub-group of lupus. Dr Hughes also noticed that pregnancies amongst lupus patients who did not have the antibody had a lower incidence of miscarriage.

An even greater discovery was just around the corner. In the early 1980s Dr Hughes and his team confirmed their belief that the antibodies were also present in patients who did not have lupus. This meant it was far more common in the wider population then they had first thought. Initially the disease was called primary antiphospholipid syndrome. The discovery received enormous international acclaim and was later renamed Hughes syndrome in honour of the doctor behind this pioneering work.

What is lupus? It is an autoimmune disease mainly affecting women – nine of ten cases are female. It is most common amongst women of childbearing age, but men and children can have it as well. Although there is limited public awareness of the disease, it is estimated that in high-risk groups (i.e. women of childbearing age with a positive family history of autoimmune disease) it can affect as many as 1 in every 200 people and is more common than MS and leukaemia. Symptoms include: chronic fatigue, joint and muscle pains, blood abnormalities, skin rashes, migraine, depression, heart or kidney failure, neurological problems and chest pain. No one knows what causes lupus but it is thought genetics play a part. It is an incurable disease and until recent years life expectancy was poor. Now with a new generation of treatments the disease can be controlled and the majority of sufferers live a relatively normal life between flare-ups.

Without doubt there is an overlap between lupus and Hughes syndrome. Tests show that 20 per cent of lupus patients have the antiphospholipid antibody. What isn't known yet is how many people suffer from Hughes syndrome alone. It could be as many as one in every two hundred people in high-risk groups. Because the discovery of the syndrome was as a result of work with lupus patients the majority of early cases made this connection between the two diseases. In the past ten years or so that perception has changed because more people are being diagnosed as having only Hughes syndrome. It is still going to take time to separate the two conditions. These autoimmune diseases are quite different. Lupus affects women primarily, whereas Hughes syndrome is more evenly distributed between the sexes. Another important difference is that lupus sufferers can go on to develop Hughes syndrome but it is extremely rare to see it happen the other way round. If you have 'sticky blood' you are unlikely to suffer at a later date from lupus.

There is still a lot of confusion about the two conditions and their association both within the medical field and amongst the general public. In America for instance 'sticky blood' is most commonly referred to as APS – antiphospholipid syndrome; there are plenty of websites that talk about APS. If you look up Hughes syndrome on the internet there are few websites to date. With growing awareness this will change. The confusion is felt by many patients: some have been told they have lupus and years later are told they also have 'sticky blood'. It is a common chain of events, the upshot is distressing for people who have to grasp the implications of not one but two complex diseases. These people are often those who have had years of illness, some joke saying they've taken so many drugs they rattle like a pillbox. There is no 'quick-fix' in these cases. One of the best things a patient can do is learn as much as he or she can about both conditions and be determined to fight them. This is often easier said than done.

Karen David

'As far back as I can remember I have had aches and pains. I recall my mom taking me to the doctor and he told me I had growing pains. I was always anaemic, had colds, flu and pneumonia at odd times during the year. I always had trouble with heavy bleeding during my period and later at numerous surgeries for endometriosis. I would then go through spells of feeling fine, only to start with the pains and infections over and over.'

Karen David, from Jackson, Tennessee has struggled with a lifetime of ill health. As with the majority of patients in the Hughes syndrome 'limbo' her road to diagnosis was tortuously long and difficult, affecting most of her adult life. She got there in the end only to find she didn't have one major illness, but two.

'In 1988 at 23 years old, I had my first pregnancy. It was very rough, I was sick the whole time and finally had an emergency Caesarean section and had my son Will. He was six weeks premature. He died the next day, his lungs had not developed and he had heart and kidney failure. It was a tough time. My husband Scott and I were grieving and then I began to get sick again. Over the next four years I suffered three miscarriages and two ectopic pregnancies. Finally at 27 I had a hysterectomy.

'The next year we adopted our son Luke. I began to feel a bit better but when Luke was one year old all the trouble began again. I started running a fever every day, I had severe fatigue, achy joints, chest pain and a terrible rash on my face and arms. In the mornings when I got up I would be so tired before I even left for work I would be in tears by 9.00 a.m. I just couldn't go on.

'Finally, after seeing doctor after doctor, I was diagnosed with lupus in 1995. By this point I couldn't even walk from the pain in my legs. The muscles and joints in my legs felt as though I had been standing on my feet for three straight months with concrete blocks attached. I had pneumonia every other month, my face was numb and I had headaches.

I don't think there was one body part that didn't hurt. When I was diagnosed with lupus the doctor said I had gone undiagnosed for nearly ten years. Even after starting the steroids, immunosup-pressives and other medications, I suffered daily. Finally I had to quit work as a dental assistant, I couldn't stay in a normal routine. I was being admitted to hospital every few months. My doctor sent me to The Johns Hopkins Hospital in Baltimore, Maryland.

'The specialist I saw there, Dr Michelle Petri, diagnosed me with APS or Hughes syndrome. She was great, she started me on warfarin and antiplatelet medication as I had numerous TIAs as well as DVTs and one pulmonary embolism. Since then it has been difficult to keep my INR regulated. When it falls below 3.0 I start to have numbness in my face, left arm and leg. I also have severe migraine, slurred speech, confusion and memory problems.

'It is so frustrating especially when you are taking the

medications to control this disease and you still suffer if your INR is not exactly where it should be. There is so little information about this condition in the USA and it is hard to get your doctor's attention on thinning your blood more so that the symptoms will improve. After months of confusion, pain, numbness, hospitalization and feeling as if I was going crazy I started my own research on this condition.

'I found Dr Graham Hughes and the Hughes Syndrome Foundation website. When I read the information on this it was like reading my whole life story. After you drive down a road that you drive daily only to realize you are lost, and you look at yourself in the mirror and you don't even recognize your own face, you become frightened. At that point you are ready to go and do whatever you can to get help. One day my son who was eight said "Mom you need to have your brain rewinded". I decided it was time to get more involved and do something. I made an appointment with Dr Hughes.

'Now, being from America I knew it would be costly to travel to London, England to see a doctor. Being out of the country my health insurance wouldn't pay and then there was the flight, hotel and food etc. It was going to be expensive. I made the appointment and just went on faith that if it was meant for me to get to London and to see Dr Hughes then God would provide a way. I got my appointment date and began to pray.

'God listened. All my friends from high school, college and my family had a fundraiser to help me get the money I needed to see Dr Hughes. I knew it would be expensive to travel, having an illness is so expensive anyway. Even with insurance in the USA you have to pay for doctor's visits and medications, hospital stays, tests, and so on.

'My friends had this huge fundraiser for me in our small community of Camden, Tennessee where we grew up. It was wonderful and they raised enough money to get me to London and back. I can't tell you what a gift it was, to see Dr Hughes and meet his staff and know they truly care about their patients' wellbeing. You take a look at the lupus pregnancy clinic with a success rate of over 70 per cent now. That makes me so proud and it brings such hope to so many women. There is hope not only in that area but in all the many areas affected by lupus and Hughes syndrome. We still have to endure the terrible pain, the side-effects of medication and the ups and downs of feeling crazy, but there is help out there.

'The great thing about seeing Dr Hughes was that he has such a great knowledge in this area. He suggested a new treatment option which included home testing and getting heparin injections. This has given me great hope as it means I have a few more good days each month. It keeps my blood more regulated and has made me feel better.

'I only wish there was more awareness from the community and from doctors who just don't understand. They can't understand how frustrating our daily life is, how you once could do normal things so easily and then suddenly you can't remember how to spell words correctly or even how to open a door! When most people come to a door the automatic reflex is to turn the handle and open it. When your brain is in a fog you have to actually stop at that door and try to think what it is you are supposed to do, it just doesn't come to you automatically. Then you get the right treatment, your blood is regulated, the fog lifts and once again you can open that door just like everyone else.'

Edwina Sewell

When Edwina sent her story to me she recommended I sat down with a large gin and tonic before I started reading. It was sound advice.

Despite repeated illnesses in her early years, Edwina qualified as a dental nurse; she trained as a civilian with the Royal Army Dental Corps. Perhaps it was a childhood in front of doctors for a variety of ailments that made her feel at home with the smell of anaesthetic and the sight of blood.

Edwina was a sickly baby and her early years were dogged with strange illnesses. When she was eight she developed herpes zoster, commonly known as shingles. Her GP had never seen it in one so young. 'From the age of eight onwards my health was never right. My mother was always being told I had growing pains, or a bug or a virus. The migraines were a frequent occurrence. My mother was told she was fussing too much, she knew something was wrong but she was made to feel stupid and ignorant.'

In her early teens Edwina had rheumatic fever after a severe throat infection. She was treated for a heart murmur and a racing pulse. 'I knew my health would never be normal again. I always seemed to be unwell. I couldn't keep up with my friends, I would come home from school exhausted and have to go to bed. My education suffered and I recall the frequent migraines which regularly made me absent from school.

'In 1973 I was bitten by an insect and reacted so badly I was rushed to hospital. I had a rash that persisted for several weeks and seemed much worse when I had been exposed to the sun.'

Edwina's ill health persisted with a bout of glandular fever and erratic periods. When she was 22, in 1980, she developed severe pain in her eyes. At the same time she began to lose control of her speech. 'I remember I was taken to the local police station on one occasion and accused of being intoxicated. My speech was slurred and I had enormous trouble trying to explain to the police that I was not drunk. I couldn't find the right words, to make things worse my balance was affected, too. I recovered within an hour, leaving the police rather puzzled at my recovery and me very worried about my symptoms.

'In the summer of 1980 I saw a neurologist because of the persistent eye pain I had been having, I was also losing the sensation in my legs and having severe migraines. He thought I had a brain tumour but nothing showed up on the brain scan. There were further investigations but they found nothing, no diagnosis was made, and I was told my symptoms were all in my head. I swore I would never see the neurologist again. I decided to forget my health problems and get on with my life.

'My job took me to Cardiff where I helped set up a new dental practice so I was working long hours. I was very tired. I had a massive attack of herpes simplex, more commonly known as cold sores. This was to be the first of many attacks that would trouble me for years to come. The virus made me very ill, it seemed to trigger off the neurological problems again, it was so bad I could not work. I lost the job I loved and had to move back to my parents' house.

'In 1982 I had a general anaesthetic for a dental operation. I reacted badly and a few weeks later I had a secondary infection that did not respond to heavy-duty antibiotics. They admitted me to hospital as I became very unwell. Overnight I became weak down one side of my body, I had visual loss in one eye. Once again I was referred to a neurologist.'

Edwina was told she had MS. Later that year she was admitted to hospital again and put on large doses of steroids. Her eyesight had become so bad she was registered partially sighted; she left the hospital in a wheelchair as she was too fatigued to walk. Over time the steroids seemed to help, and Edwina managed to return to work part-time, but the unpredictability of her condition, in particular more frequent migraine, forced her to retire in 1984.

'Over the next few years I had a few funny turns but my parents and I questioned the diagnosis of MS because I did not do what the textbooks said. I was investigated for epilepsy, but the tests were negative. I developed frightening mood swings that hit me out of the blue. I had episodes of slurred speech, confusion and weakness in my limbs. The doctors said these were common complications of MS. I was convinced I was imagining the symptoms.

'I continued to doubt the diagnosis then one morning towards the end of 1988 I woke up to find I was weak down the right side of my body. My right hand and arm were badly affected. A local GP gave me a high-dose steroid injection; the neurologist said the MS had relapsed. But I realized I had suffered a peripheral nerve palsy in my arm, which MS does not cause as it attacks the central nervous system. I told my GP, but he still insisted I had MS.' Edwina changed GP, but got the same verdict – she had MS.

'A few more years passed and my life became intolerable. My health was deteriorating but the doctors would not listen to me or my parents. It was now very obvious to me that my symptoms could not be due to MS but I began to doubt my own judgement. I started to think I should accept the diagnosis although I knew in my heart it was wrong.

'In 1991 I noticed pain in my hip. It became impossible to walk and I found myself in hospital undergoing tests. They found I had avascular necrosis (crumbling of the hip joint). The orthopaedic surgeon I saw questioned the diagnosis of MS but was overruled by my GP and neurologist. No one even mentioned to me that this problem with my hip could have been caused by the prolonged use of steroids.'

Over the next few years Edwina retreated to her bedroom, she was virtually housebound. She was sick and disillusioned with a medical profession that couldn't, or wouldn't, find out what was really wrong with her.

In 1993 she developed swollen joints and was admitted to hospital. Septic arthritis was diagnosed. This was treated with antibiotics but she went on to have severe chest pains. They found Edwina had pleurisy and pericarditis (inflammation of the lining around the heart).

'About this time I had a very abnormal reaction to the sun. I was sitting in the garden one afternoon when I noticed a rash on my exposed skin. This started to form into very tiny blisters and I started to swell up. An hour later I was very uncomfortable – and worried about my appearance.

'The next day I was due to see my consultant, he immediately sent me for emergency treatment; for the first time lupus was mentioned. I had never even heard of it.

'I had an MRI scan which confirmed I definitely did not have MS and never had had MS. I wanted an apology from the doctors who put me through absolute hell for the past ten years, I have been on an emotional roller-coaster. And now I had no name for my symptoms. Although I never believed I had MS, at least I had a name; now there was no label, what did I say if people asked what was wrong with me?

'My consultant was certain I had lupus but the tests proved him wrong. They did find I had a connective tissue disease, of which I was told there were many.

'I spent the next three years with no diagnosis and no treatment. My health continued to deteriorate and I hit an all-time low. Nobody seemed to understand how I needed a label for my symptoms, I needed a diagnosis, I needed to know what I was fighting.'

Edwina was admitted to hospital on a number of occasions at this time. At one stage she was so ill she lost consciousness and her parents were told to expect the worst. But she pulled through. The list of symptoms was daunting:

- migraine
- vertigo
- fatigue
- chest/joint/muscle pain
- hair loss
- partial deafness
- memory loss

- confusion
- visual disturbances
- hearing voices.

It was by chance that Edwina got on the road to a diagnosis. While she was visiting her parents, who had moved away, she hurt her back. She saw an orthopaedic surgeon who heard her medical history and said she must have lupus. When she said her blood test was negative he told her she could still have lupus.

'I went home and visited the library, I saw a copy of *The Lupus Book* by Daniel Wallace. He stated in black and white that it was possible to misdiagnose MS for lupus and it was also possible to diagnose lupus with a negative blood test. That same week my mother and I watched Dr Graham Hughes talking about lupus on television. Everything he said seemed to relate to me. We couldn't believe what we were hearing. I knew I had to get referred to Dr Hughes.

'I saw him six months later. He diagnosed lupus, Sjögren's syndrome and possible Hughes syndrome. He didn't hesitate, and above all he understood how ill I felt and the fight I had had to reach his door. The relief was absolutely overwhelming, I had a name for all my symptoms! They could all be explained and, for the first time, they all made sense. I was not imagining my symptoms and I certainly wasn't crazy.'

But getting the treatment right took time. Edwina reacted badly to a number of the medications, and the anti-inflammatory drug azathioprine caused liver problems. It also transpired that the years without a diagnosis had taken their toll.

'It was apparent that the great delay in obtaining the correct diagnosis had caused irreversible damage to my body. I have severe calcinosis [a deposit of calcium, in Edwina's case in her muscles]. This affects my mobility and has left me with a gait that has to be seen to be believed. The calcinosis and prolonged use of steroids has also caused muscle wastage which also affect my mobility.

'In 1998 I was put on methotrexate and that made a vast difference to the joint pains and some of the other lupus symptoms. I was able to maintain a reasonable state of health if I stayed on low-dose steroids, plaquenil, methotrexate and low-dose aspirin. However, I still found my life was being controlled by the endless migraines, confusion, memory loss, visual disturbances and weird brain fug which made me lose track of time.

'In September last year [2001] I started taking warfarin, and I have to say I have never looked back. My life has improved so much I can now say that I have a life – not just an existence. Within weeks of starting this treatment I was able to shower and dress every day for the first time in about twenty years. To any healthy individual this may sound crazy but to me it was a huge achievement.

'It has been difficult to maintain the correct INR; without any doubt if it drops below 3.5 all my symptoms return. But I could not have considered writing this if I was not taking warfarin. I would have typed the wrong letters, I would not have had the concentration, I would have not even got out of my bed if I had a migraine or brain fug.

'It hurts terribly if I look back and think what could have been if I had received the correct diagnosis years ago. My health stopped me from getting married and having children. My career was cut short. My family have sacrificed so much to let me have some degree of independence. And financially, life is an endless struggle. But I continue to take each day as it comes. I have to pace myself if I am to keep some control over the fatigue which, in hindsight, is much better than it used to be. I have learnt not to ignore symptoms and I ask for help when I know I am heading for a flare up. I know I can now cope with my condition much better because I do not have the persistent migraines and confusion. If my mobility would improve that would be an added bonus. If the pleurisy and pericarditis disappeared permanently it would be a double bonus.

'I find the ignorance about both lupus and Hughes syndrome appalling. I attend a local hospital anticoagulant clinic where they admitted they had never heard of Hughes syndrome. I am one of the fortunate ones who has been diagnosed and treated. I hope my experiences will help others who are still striving for the correct diagnosis.'

10

The Rest of the Body

No part of the body is safe from Hughes syndrome, from the tips of your toes to the top of your head. Each patient has his own set of symptoms; no two people are completely alike. The nature of the condition, namely that it affects the blood, means it recognizes no boundaries. So far this broader aspect of the disease is still relatively uncharted territory. But as more people are diagnosed with Hughes syndrome there is a growing evidence of the impact it can have on less obvious parts of the body.

Beverley Sparrow

Beverley Sparrow first learnt she had something wrong with her blood when she became a donor. Six months after giving blood in 1982 she was told they had found an abnormality and sent her for tests. The doctors said she might be in the early stages of lupus, but she never got a firm diagnosis.

'Two years later I started to have a pain in my right foot. My GP referred me to a consultant. I was 34 at the time. I noticed one toe on my foot was going blue. The professor didn't make much of it, I wasn't sent for more investigations, just sent home. For the next twelve months my toe got worse, it was incredibly painful. I had been complaining for such a long time to the doctors without them doing anything about it I thought maybe it was in my head.

'Then in May 1985 I was finally referred to a vascular surgeon. I was sent for arteriogram. The surgeon phoned me at home with the result of the test and said it showed I had a total occlusion or blockage of the main artery to my leg. He said he didn't know if he could save my leg. I was in utter shock. I went to hospital for the operation that was meant to unblock the artery. I was so unwell after that, I reacted badly to the anaesthetic. Then my foot got worse, all my toes turned black. In June they said they couldn't save the toes, they had become black and slimy. They were amputated. I wasn't told the foot had gangrene until after the operation.

'Still things got worse, my foot didn't heal, the gangrene had spread. In the following September I had a further operation. This time half my foot was chopped off in what they called a "guillotine amputation" where it is literally cut in a straight line. They said they had to do this to stop the gangrene spreading up my leg.

'After the last operation my foot didn't heal, it went completely black. I became very ill, I was in hospital for a long time. I couldn't understand why I was becoming so sick, I lost lots of weight, went down to $8^1/_2$ stone (54 kg). Rather than getting better I started to have gangrenous lesions on my left foot. Both my feet were bandaged. Worst of all they couldn't control the pain as the morphine and methadone didn't work for me. Words cannot describe the pain.

'I was never told anything, I didn't have a diagnosis. One day I lay there and thought "If I don't get out of this hospital I am going to die". I got into my wheelchair and asked the nurse if I was dying, I didn't get a clear answer so I discharged myself. They tried to stop me but I knew I had to get out of there. I called a friend who took me home.'

Beverley had a good district nurse who visited her at home and helped with the painful dressings. But Beverley's ordeal was far from over. Her feet did not heal and she went for a check-up with the vascular surgeon in March 1986.

'My ankle joint had seized up so I had developed what they call drop foot, where you can't lift or control your foot. The consultant had reviewed my case and told me the right foot would never heal and I had to have my leg amputated below the knee. He had already arranged a bed for me in the hospital. I was in complete shock again but there was no way I was going to let them take my leg. I refused to have the amputation, instead I saw my local GP near Alton in Hampshire where I live.

'Her name is Dr Margaret Hall and she saved my life. Dr Hall had gone through my notes and put the various pieces of the picture together. She had heard of Dr Graham Hughes and his work at St Thomas', she knew about antiphospholipid antibodies. She got me an appointment to see Dr Hughes. He gave me the diagnosis I needed so badly, in those days it was called antiphospholipid syndrome, now Hughes syndrome. I had never heard of it. I was put on warfarin and low-dose aspirin. The drugs worked and at last I began to get better.

'Dr Hughes didn't comment about how long it had taken for

me to get a diagnosis, what he did say was he just wished he had seen me sooner. My amputated foot was a mess and I had to have three operations to remove protruding bone, I also had skin grafts. My foot finally healed in 1987. It was then I started the long road of learning to walk again. I began driving an automatic car the next year; now I drive a manual. I am 52 years old and work full-time as a voluntary driver for the social services.

'What all this taught me is doctors don't know everything, patients can tell if something is wrong with them. If you aren't happy with your treatment and you don't get a diagnosis you have to keep on fighting until you do.'

Carol Smith

At 40 Carol Smith has a busy life. She juggles caring for her two young children with running the family business managing two service stations and going to college. Carol has a strong positive approach to life and she believes it is that attitude that kept her going when she became seriously ill seven years ago. She was pregnant with her second child Charlie when the sight in one of her eyes began to weaken. 'Looking through my left eye things had become all brownish, a bit like the dried blood you see on a microscope slide, there were brown lines and lumps across everything I looked at.

'I went to see my local optician who was wonderful and thorough. After looking into my eyes he said I should get in my car and drive straight to the casualty unit at Maidstone Hospital as something was clearly wrong. He had seen what they call "floaters" in my eye. Apparently the vision blurs because the eye fills up with these tiny clots of blood. I went to casualty. They detected lupus in my blood and I was referred to the lupus clinic at St Thomas'.'

The doctors believed the problem with her eyes was not connected. 'They were insistent there wasn't a link between lupus and my acute retinal vasculitis but I felt sure there must be. I couldn't believe that two things were going on at the same time and were totally separate.'

As the months passed the sight in her left eye got worse, to the point where Carol could see nothing with it, then her other eye started to lose vision as well. At one point the doctors told Carol that she was virtually blind.

She was seeing a consultant ophthalmologist who was puzzled as to why Carol's eyes were not responding well to treatment. The consultant knew Dr Hughes and asked him for his opinion. His view was Carol had 'sticky blood' and should be treated with anticoagulants.

'The effect of the warfarin was remarkable. Within a few days I had my eyesight back, I was amazed and obviously delighted.'

Carol is back to her busy life and although she still has some reduced vision her eyesight is almost completely normal.

Frances Simner

Frances Simner was teaching a biology class when suddenly all she could see were hands and tabletops but nothing above that level. This was in 1987.

'It had been a normal day, I was teaching from a raised rostrum in an old-fashioned school science laboratory. I looked at the class and realized the top half of my vision had gone in both eyes. All I could see were the hands of the students on the desks and the desk tops. I couldn't see their upper bodies or the top part of the room, that part of my vision was a haze, it was all beige coloured. I asked one of the students to come and look at my eyes because I couldn't see. Fortunately they were a super group of sixth-formers and were very helpful. The episode lasted a few minutes then it cleared and my normal vision came back. It was a terrifying experience.

'I went to see a doctor at the local hospital, Queen Mary's in Sidcup. They examined me and said I was fine, I was told to take some aspirin and to go home.

'This loss of vision continued for the next 14 years. It was intermittent, sometimes one eye, rarely both. Usually it was like a finger across the visual field or approximately half the eye lost vision. These episodes lasted anything between one and twenty minutes and initially occurred several times each day. I continued to teach, I just got on with things. I had no other symptoms for years, just the problem with my vision but that would come and go.'

But Frances did have to give up teaching in school in 1994 because she had developed a severe headache. 'It was horrendous, the headache started in May and carried on to the end of July. I went to sleep with it and woke up with it.' No treatment from her

GP had any effect on the headache. The headaches came and went after that.

'I found as I got older I needed glasses and so began seeing an optician. She knew of these episodes when I lost part of my vision; she was concerned and perplexed as she could find no answers to what was happening. In June 2000, 13 years after this began, my optician said it really was time that something was done to sort this out. I was on BUPA so I went to see an ophthalmologist privately. He said this had nothing to do with my eyes, it was to do with my heart. After that there was no let up, everyone was determined to find out what was wrong. I think I must have had every test available and because it was done under health insurance, things happened quickly. An MRI scan showed I had suffered several mini-strokes. This had done permanent damage taking 25 per cent of my visual field in both eyes.

'In April 2001 I saw Dr Hunt at St Thomas' who told me I had Hughes syndrome. I was put on warfarin but at first it was diabolical, it made my headaches much worse. It took me eight weeks to adjust to it, and now I don't get the headaches any more.'

Frances says the worst part of the condition for her is the loss of memory. She has discovered that the mini-strokes have left large holes in the part of her brain that holds memories.

'The thing that came to light was the extent of my loss, it is huge. My husband Barry and I have been together since we were teenagers. We are very close and happy doing everything together. These days Barry acts as my memory because I have lost so much.

'In 2000 we were guests at the men's tennis semi-finals at Wimbledon. We had lunch, on the table next to us was Bruce Forsyth, the sun was shining and it was a brilliant day. But I have no recollection of it, nothing at all. If you asked me about it I would say I had never been to Wimbledon. I only know about it because Barry has told me. When I look at a photo of it, it's like a picture in a magazine, it is like I am looking at complete strangers.

'I do find this terribly distressing, we have taken lots of photos over the years and I use those to put the bits of my life back together. Before the diagnosis of Hughes syndrome I knew I had a poor memory but I was adept at hiding it, now Barry insists I tell him if I really can remember something or not.

'The memory loss never seemed to affect my ability to teach, perhaps because course programmes are very structured, and repeated many times. I continue to teach now, part-time and to adults. I do get sudden blanks; a few months ago I was standing in front of a class and in mid-sentence I couldn't remember what I was talking about, nothing was coming out of my mouth and if I did manage to say anything it was gibberish. I told the class to take a break, I waited for the episode to pass and then carried on. I think there is no point weeping and wailing about this, that just wouldn't do any good. I just get on with my life.'

11

The Fight for Diagnosis

One feature of 'sticky blood' that crops up time and again is the difficulty people have getting a diagnosis. Of all those I have interviewed for this book not one had a straightforward path to finding out what was wrong with them. Most often it was quite the opposite: they had a terrible struggle to get answers and the right treatment. A few did have the good fortune to come across more enlightened doctors who kept up to speed with the latest news in medicine so they knew what Hughes syndrome was. Sadly, at the present time those doctors are few and far between.

Many people go through months and often years of uncertainty before they discover what the mystery illness is that has ruined their health. Once again most people I have spoken to talked of getting to the point where they felt they might be going mad or perhaps they were becoming hypochondriacs. In defence of the doctors, it is fair to say 'sticky blood' affects people in so many different ways no two cases are alike. This makes diagnosis very difficult. I found it interesting that quite a few people discovered what was wrong by searching the internet. There are growing numbers of people who meet up in cyberspace (see p. 89 for websites) and compare notes on 'sticky blood', like an informal club or forum. It is a phenomenon that has evolved without preconception or plan but through the sheer need of so many to know more. It is also quite telling that people are not prepared to accept a diagnosis if they think it is wrong.

In the cases where people have been diagnosed with lupus it is slightly easier to expose the antiphospholipid antibodies: the patient already has a recognized autoimmune disease and so blood is tested regularly. But the majority of people start from square one and that is hard. It is quite common for patients to have been seen by a string of consultants in a variety of medical specialisms over a period of many years but still be in the dark about what is making them so ill. The diversity of symptoms has confused the picture and left doctors puzzled and unable to provide patients with the answers they need. Many of those who do get the diagnosis and find themselves in front of specialists of Dr Hughes' calibre are the ones who have a combination of determination and luck, they are those who shout the loudest. It has often taken time but they get there in the end. This is great for them, but 'sticky blood' is very common, and if Dr Hughes is right, it will eclipse other autoimmune diseases in the years to come. So where are all the other sufferers of 'sticky blood'? A widely held fear is that those who are too ill to fight or have difficulty shouting are being overlooked. How many people with MS actually don't have MS but Hughes syndrome instead? Then there are those who have suffered terrible migraine for years when a correct diagnosis could have dealt with that pain. What about patients who have been told they have early dementia and do not? Or the women who keep losing their babies through miscarriage for the sake of the right diagnosis and some low-dose aspirin? It is a disturbing thought that there are tens, hundreds, probably even thousands of people who are struggling with terrible symptoms without knowing what is wrong; people writing themselves off as hypochondriacs, gradually becoming more ill as the disease attacks and remains untreated. These people are not getting the help available; for the sake of an inexpensive blood test and readily available drugs they suffer in silence.

Perhaps the stories of those who were heard in the end will help show them the way.

Ann McFall

Ann says she had a headache for eighteen years. Hard to believe but almost every day of her life after the birth of her son she was plagued with various degrees of pain in her head. And the older she got the worse it was. No matter what tests were carried out and which consultant she saw doctors could find nothing wrong. The results were all negative. For Ann the frustration turned to depression and the fear that she was imagining the symptoms.

'Think what it would be like if as soon as you opened your eyes in the morning you got this pain all over your eyes like a terrible hangover; it made you feel so bad that you had to run to the toilet to be sick, and worse still, no painkillers worked. That was what it was like for me for years since my son was born in 1983. The only thing I could do was lie on the bed with a damp cloth over my eyes but then I couldn't sleep for the pain. It was horrible. I think my poor husband must have got sick of my moaning on about how bad my head was. It made me so bad-tempered with everyone, I couldn't be myself.'

Ann comes from Rotherhithe in south-east London and is 39; she spent almost half her life trying to find out what was wrong in the hope she could stop the pain.

'After my Ryan was born I was quite sick and no one knew why. I had headache and joint pains. At one point they thought something was wrong with my liver. My skin started to go blotchy. I was in and out of hospital for tests but they all came back negative. In the end I felt I must be neurotic, I was convinced they would all think I was one of those hypochondriacs. My GP was very concerned about me and I was given some special migraine medicine.

'In 1990 they did find something in my blood, at long last. They said it was something that showed I had rheumatism but now I know it was more likely lupus. I am not sure what they planned to do because all of that was put to one side when I fell pregnant.

'The pregnancy was a disaster. I lost my baby at six months. I kept saying to the doctors I didn't feel well and I knew there was something wrong. Tests had shown my thyroid wasn't working and I went to my GP who said they would keep a close eye on me. 'My waters broke early and we went to hospital. The doctor there said they must get the baby out, he said they would put me on a drip to make it quick but instead it took 24 hours. The baby was dead. They laid it near me and then took it away. I was hysterical, I was beside myself.

'After that I was very ill. They thought I had blood poisoning, all my symptoms became a hundred times worse. I think it was after losing my baby that the lupus really kicked in. My GP at the time was brilliant. She did keep a close watch on me and in the end she thought something dodgy was going on. It was when I was having my daughter in 1993 that she got me a referral to the lupus pregnancy clinic at St Thomas' Hospital. 'I was monitored closely, it was a difficult pregnancy but my little girl, Ellie, is now eight so something must have gone right.'

Afterwards the headaches became even more ferocious and Ann developed other symptoms. She had numbness in her fingers, toes and parts of her face, known as peripheral neuropathy. Her joints were swollen and her skin was covered in rashes. She had chronic fatigue and flu-like symptoms with a high temperature.

'My skin would get so bad I wouldn't leave the house, I would stay indoors and cry. If I did go out young children would look at my skin and ask if I had cancer.

'In September 2000 I saw Dr Hughes and he did some more tests which confirmed I had 'sticky blood' as well as lupus. He put me on warfarin. It was so nice to talk to a doctor who understood what I had, he didn't make me feel I was mad. He would ask me if I had a certain symptom and when I said "Yes" he would calmly nod his head. It was great because he knew what I was going through. I thought "Oh, thank God, this is someone who believes me."

'Within two weeks the headaches had gone, it was heaven. Suddenly it was a pleasure to get up in the morning, I didn't have the pain and so I wasn't grumpy with the kids. I did wonder if it was true, if the pain would come back. I do still get the occasional headache but nothing like what I used to suffer. When Dr Hughes saw me he said I had no quality of life because of the pain I was suffering and he said the treatment would change that. He was right, I do now have a good quality of life and I am grateful for each day that passes without a headache.

'I really hope and pray that people are made aware of both conditions – lupus and Hughes syndrome. I think there must be a lot of people out there who don't know they have these conditions. Before I knew what I had, I felt, at times, that I wanted to die; once I knew what was wrong I no longer felt like a freak. It was such a relief.'

Kate Welch

Young people never expect to become ill, so Kate Welch was staggered when she ended up in hospital with a clot in her right calf at the age of 32. A successful systems analyst in Chicago, Illinois, Kate had never been seriously unwell. She had just got married and was a highly motivated career woman.

'Three months before the clot happened I had been to see a doctor because I just didn't feel right. I was under a lot of stress. At work there was a company merger and I was newly married. My heart would race and then beat strangely. I was totally exhausted for no reason at times, and my vision started to go. I generally felt light-headed and dizzy. On top of all that I couldn't seem to concentrate on things the way I used to.

'Despite this I didn't feel the outside events in my life should have made me feel so bad. I have always been a high-energy career-motivated "take on the world" kind of person. So after doing some tests, including heart imaging, lung scan and basic blood examinations, my doctor determined I probably had costochondritis, which is an inflammation of the cartilage between the ribs. He told me to take it easy and said the rib pain would probably stop soon. It was only later I found out costochondritis is an autoimmune condition.

'So three months later on 7 April 2000, I was checked into the hospital with the clot. I felt my doctor was totally incompetent and never even ran the right tests. It took three months to find this out because my records were lost by both her and the hospital. Also, when I asked about support stockings she said I didn't need them, and she wanted to take me off Coumadin [warfarin] after only three months. When I said I wanted to stay on longer, she said, "What will people think?", as if that mattered! In any case, I searched the internet and learned so much. I was able to find out what tests were supposed to be run and then in August I found another doctor who agreed to run some of the right tests. And voilà! I was positive for anticardiolipin antibodies.

'My current doctor is much better. He is also a haematologist, so he understands a lot more about the problem. But, I have to say, he still does not seem to associate the APS or Hughes syndrome with any of my "stress" symptoms.

'Whenever I would say I just didn't feel right he would dismiss it as stress. It wasn't until I found the Forum, a website on the internet, and read about other peoples' symptoms and day-to-day lives with the disease that I finally understood why I was feeling so strange. Looking back, I can see that the "stress" symptoms were actually the beginnings of the syndrome. I also now know that the symptoms are not necessarily all because of stress, and that I am not going crazy or just being a hypochondriac! It is a very real part of the disease and I believe it is one of the things doctors know least about.

'As for what impact "sticky blood" has had on my life you could say it has "rocked my world". I am so lucky to have an understanding spouse and supportive parents, but life as I knew it will never be the same. I used to be full of life, out-going, popular, career-motivated, nothing could stand in my way and I loved my life. I am now anxious, afraid, lonely, my self-confidence waxes and wanes, and I have gained weight. Between the employment uncertainty and my health uncertainty I have not been able to finish my master's degree course and I fear I may never get it done. I am also registered to take the PE (professional engineers) exam, but I cannot fathom how I will be able to work full-time and study. In the past, this would not have fazed me. Now, I am just exhausted all the time, and have little enthusiasm for most things. However, I do consider myself lucky as far as my work goes. I am currently able to go to the doctor whenever I need to, and can run out for INR blood tests easily.

'Managing the disease once I was diagnosed became a major part of my life: getting regular blood tests, changing my diet, no drinking. Then there's the time spent looking for answers from different doctors and on the internet: trying to connect with other people who feel as I do, and trying to make some sense of why this happened when I was perfectly healthy before.

'Another huge impact has been the issue of having children. Pregnancy is very uncertain and requires shots and no one can predict the impact of the disease on the foetus. Then there's also the increased risk of me developing another life-threatening clot.

'My biggest concern is with the hereditary considerations of the disease. The current literature says it is not genetic, but "tends to run in families". So my husband and I are worried about whether we should risk having children of our own; we thought it might be better to adopt. It is so depressing for me and I feel I couldn't bear the thought of another human being going through this.

'We looked closely at our family history, certainly autoimmune conditions did not seem to run in my family. My mother did have a clot a few days after I was born.

'Although she is factor V Leiden-positive, she has never been on anticoagulant therapy (except for the first 6 months after her clot) and has not had any problems since. Now she is a very healthy 74-year-old. Luckily, she did not pass the factor V gene on to me. We also went to the University of Chicago Hospitals for a genetic counselling session. We spoke with the head of the department and she did not feel that this was a hereditary condition, and that I should go ahead and have children and not worry about it. My primary-care doctor and my gynaecologist also did not see any reason not to have children. I am still concerned, but we traced the family history and there really does not seem to be any evidence of Hughes syndrome or any other autoimmune problems. So, we are going to proceed with trying to have one or two children of our own. I am really dreading the shots, and am trying to get myself into as good physical condition as I can before we even start down the pregnancy path.

'My condition is stable and I wear full-height compression stockings. I get my INR checked once a month and am learning to accept my new life. I am trying to exercise regularly and lose some weight, but it's really hard because I'm so tired most of the time, but I will get there in the end.'

Carole Judge

Carole, who's 54 and lives in Coventry in the west Midlands, has strong feelings about the current lack of awareness of Hughes syndrome. After what she and many others have been through Carole believes there should be a media campaign on television, radio and in the press to let people know about 'sticky blood'. She feels if more of the public and doctors knew of the condition there would be a lot less unnecessary suffering.

'I used to work as a catering manager at a college of further education but I had to retire two years ago because of ill health. I have several conditions; they include Raynaud's, which I have had since I was a child, fibromyalgia, which was diagnosed five years ago, lupus, Sjögren's and recently I discovered I had Hughes syndrome.

'In 1991 I was taken ill on a holiday in the USA. I had an allergic reaction to the sun and I also had a gastric viral attack. I was having lots of different health difficulties: kidney problems, irritable bowel symptoms, joint pains, fatigue, skin rashes, couldn't sleep. I gained weight, although my eating habits had not changed. I developed memory problems, it was like being dyslexic with words and numbers. I would start to write the next word before I had finished the one I was on. I found I could not remember names of people I had worked with for a long time, or procedures I had operated for many years.

'Now I have a number of symptoms; TIAs [mini-strokes], patches of skin that are red and get larger – sometimes going septic – red spots on my fingers and my kidney function is deteriorating.

'I was told by two specialists to see someone else, I was told by another specialist that it was all in my mind and to "go home and have some aromatherapy". Because of what that doctor wrote on my hospital notes my GP wanted to put me on tranquillizers and would not believe I was ill. So I changed my GP. But that doctor's view was still on my notes so when I was admitted into hospital in 2001 and started having TIAs the specialist I was under did not believe me and would not treat me. She also told me to see someone else. If it was not for my family I would have thought it was my imagination, I got angry that nobody seemed to help me or want to help me.

'The turning point was Dr Hughes, that simple. He listened to me, he asked questions, and he believed me, he diagnosed lupus, Sjögren's and Hughes syndrome. The relief was tremendous, he restored my faith in doctors.

'We need to educate the medical profession in how to listen to their patients. My new and excellent GP told me that some doctors will not admit they have no idea what is wrong with someone, so they tell the patient it is their fault or in their mind. I would like to see people talking about "sticky blood" on the television, hear them on the radio, and see posters in all GP surgeries.

'I would advise any person who has an illness but can't get a diagnosis for it is to keep on fighting, see different doctors, make a noise and stand up for yourself, remember doctors do not want to take on complicated cases.'

Depression

A worrying number of patients I have spoken to have had an extremely difficult struggle to get a diagnosis because doctors really did think their symptoms were all in their minds. These unfortunate people were written off as neurotics or hypochondriacs. They found themselves treated for depression for many years while the 'sticky blood' symptoms got worse. It is tough to stand up to doctors and say you are not depressed, or that you are depressed but because of your illness. When you are unwell it is hard to find extra energy to fight, but sadly with such an odd condition as Hughes syndrome it is when you are the most ill that you need strength to take on the medical establishment. If you don't you could be consigning yourself to years of antidepressants and a worsening physical condition.

Judi Page

For many years Judi Page was treated for depression. She complained of a wide variety of symptoms but none of them were looked at as a whole picture until recent years.

'I have not been 100 per cent fit since having glandular fever when I was 16. I got tired easily and had no stamina. But that might have been Sjögren's syndrome, which I also suffer from and was diagnosed in 2001 at the same time as the Hughes syndrome. It seems "sticky blood" is often accompanied by various other complaints.

'The problems got worse after I had pneumonia just over 14 years ago. I started getting migraine, eczema, irritable bowel syndrome, depression and a lot of fatigue. For many years doctors put it all down to depression. Then about two years ago the migraines got much worse as did the irritable bowel. Last summer I had headaches every day, many of them were incapacitating. I also fell over a few times for no apparent reason; at one point I fell down a flight of stairs.

'The doctors investigated the migraines and falls; this revealed I had something wrong with my heart. I was diagnosed as having angina and the falls were to do with vasovagal syncope (fainting).

'As you can see from the length of time it took to find out what I was suffering from, more than 14 years, I had extreme difficulty getting a diagnosis possibly because the symptoms were put down to depression. Even after things got really bad a year ago the rheumatologist missed it. He diagnosed Sjögren's and tested me for lupus, the result was negative. He missed the antiphospholipid syndrome despite the fact I have been told more recently it should have been obvious I was suffering from this condition.

'I did some of my own research about lupus and Hughes syndrome on the internet. I decided I would see someone as a private patient. I did have a blood test for the antibodies done locally and that came back normal, so my GP wasn't convinced I had APS and once again said my problems were due to depression. At this time I had a brain MRI scan showing two small abnormalities but that was ignored.

'I saw Dr Munther Khamashta, luckily he didn't believe the blood test result from the local hospital and retested me. The level of antibodies was high. It is just as well I am persistent, I nearly gave up so many times because no one apart from a couple of friends believed me. I was so lucky to find Dr Khamashta, at long last I got a diagnosis, in November 2001.

'The impact on my life is horrific, especially as I am a freelance accountant and am single. My social life was difficult to maintain after I had pneumonia, I just didn't have enough energy to work and socialize as well. So I have only a few friends left, not everyone can cope with the illness. You never know when you will feel well enough to go out even if you take time off work in an effort to make sure you will be able to go.

'Bad days can come out of the blue, for no reason at all. I haven't been able to work at all since the end of June 2001 and for six months before that I could only manage three days a week. A few employers were very understanding, I did the hours but not necessarily on particular days.

'The upshot is I am in deep trouble financially and I am having to sell my flat in New Malden, Surrey, as I can't afford to live there much longer. With no one to support me I am very reliant on friends and neighbours to help with things like shopping. It gets very lonely at times and it certainly isn't a fun life. I find it is a constant fight even to do everyday things. It is also quite frightening to know you are prone to blood clotting, night time is the worst when there is no one around.

'I would say to others with this condition they must remember that their GP probably won't have had a patient with this before. So you have to get as much information together as you can to back you up and help you fight for a referral to a consultant who is experienced in this field.'

12

Catastrophic Antiphospholipid Syndrome

The most frightening manifestation of 'sticky blood' is something known as catastrophic antiphospholipid syndrome. Fortunately this is extremely rare but when it does happen the impact on the body is devastating. Without immediate treatment it can kill.

This condition occurs when a person who has APL suddenly develops clots all over their body. In the few cases that are documented it is not uncommon for the patient to have been generally healthy before the attack, they might not even know they have the antibody in their blood. The clots cover the whole body and can affect a few or all vital organs. Dr Hughes says this is a full-blown medical emergency, treatment needs to be speedy and aggressive to save the person's life. No one knows what causes this terrible condition, although in some patients it appears an infection is the trigger, like a virus or sore throat. Another extremely rare cause is stopping anticoagulant drug treatment in someone with Hughes syndrome.

Alan Varney

Alan Varney, an engineer, moved from South Yorkshire to the Brighton area in 1994 when he was in his early 50s. The move left him oddly tired and breathless; he was puzzled by this as he was usually energetic and felt well. He had been quite healthy most of his life other than suffering some annoying ulcers on both legs that needed pressure dressings. But this didn't bother him. He was more concerned that three months after the move he was still breathless.

'My GP thought I was asthmatic, he gave me an inhaler and told me to see him again in a week. But I was back before the week was up as I was worse. I was still going to work, which involved a lot of driving. During one trip on my way back to the office I had a sharp pain in the right side of my chest. I told no one but I must have looked unwell as one of my colleagues insisted on driving me home and and I let him; to be honest I knew I was unable to drive at that stage.

'From this point on my recollections are very hazy and I will let my wife, Marian, tell the rest of the story.'

Marian Varney recalls: 'Alan had a very bad night, he was vomiting and during the night he just wasn't himself. He lost his co-ordination and started rambling. I told him I should call an ambulance but he wouldn't have it. In the morning he couldn't walk properly, I'm not sure how I got him to the doctor. Once we were there our GP thought the problem might be neurological and got him a bed at the Royal Sussex County Hospital. No one would confirm he had suffered a stroke but that was what we both thought. The male nurse though said stroke normally affected only one side whereas Alan was having problems with co-ordination on both sides of his body. They didn't know what had made him so ill. After a week the doctors said Alan could go home for the weekend, but suddenly they changed their minds as they found a clot on his lung. Over the next 12 days Alan's feet were getting darker in colour but this did come and go. Never a day went by without a blood test and all the time Alan was obviously deteriorating.

'At one point I came into the ward and there were three consultants gathered around Alan's bed, I knew there must be something terribly wrong. They told me they had found something abnormal in his blood. It was called "antiphospholipid", I just couldn't get my head around that. I made them repeat it time and again, and then I got them to spell it out so I could write it down. I had also heard Alan might have lupus and it was by sheer luck I had noticed in the waiting room off the ward there were lots of leaflets about lupus. I had heard of that disease but had no idea what it was. On the leaflet was the address for Lupus UK. I contacted them and they sent more information about antiphospholipid syndrome. When I showed the nurses on the ward they asked for a copy as they had never heard of it before.'

Marian's feeling of foreboding having seen the team of consultants at her husband's bedside was not misplaced. Alan's legs had become gangrenous and although no one really knew what was wrong with him the decision was the legs had to be removed.

'A relative and I were visiting Alan and when we arrived there was a surgeon at the desk in the ward talking to the nurses, my companion laughed and said "Hello, it looks as though someone's for the chop"; at the time I didn't realize it was Alan. The screens were around his bed. The surgeon told me things weren't good at all and they were going to have to amputate both legs. He said whether they were cut above or below the knee depended on what they found.

'I couldn't take it in, I was in shock. I thought they might take his toes as I had seen a form by his bed that said his toes had gangrene. I knew his feet were in a terrible state. But it was clearly more serious than that.

'By now Alan was very unwell. He was in a lot of pain. His body was burning up and he was rambling again. He was glistening with sweat and he had red blotches everywhere; I now know they were hundreds of blood clots just under his skin. He was in a bad way.

'One of the doctors I had come to know told me it was unlikely Alan would survive. His kidneys had failed, his lungs were close to failing and his heart was badly affected.

'When I heard they thought he wouldn't survive the operation I had an odd reaction, I just thought I had to get out of there, I had to get home and speak to our four children. I felt guilty but I couldn't stay there any longer.

'So I went home and told the children how sick Alan was. The hospital called to say he was on his way to theatre and then we heard nothing for hours. We all expected the worst, we thought Alan was going to die. It got to six o'clock and my son said he couldn't stand the waiting any more, so he phoned. When he got through and spoke to them he started shouting that Dad was alive and in intensive care.

'We went to the hospital and my son ran up the stairs to get to the ward while the rest of us waited for the lift. When we got up there he was outside the ward and crying, he said that wasn't his Dad in there.

'The thing is Alan was 6 ft 2 in before the amputation, so in his bed with a cage over his stumps he looked so small. The nurses did move the cage down to make him look a bit better but it was hard for us all.'

Marian says no one knows how many strokes Alan suffered before the operation but once his legs were amputated he began to recover. His eyesight was affected and he still rambled but she could see a positive change in him.

'The doctors didn't know what to do with him, they were quite honest about it. One doctor in intensive care came to me and said "How do you think he is?" and I thought why ask me, you're the doctor.

'From the moment Alan's legs were removed from below the knee his recovery started. His platelet count began to rise and he was started on heparin intravenously. Later, that was changed to warfarin. In those first days in intensive care, Alan was obviously getting better.

'His real improvement came when he was allowed home. I could have a conversation with him again. A few months later he had some artificial legs made, that was the middle of July. By Christmas he was walking pretty well with the help of sticks. He has never looked back since.'

Marian was told Alan had made medical history by surviving catastrophic antiphospholipid syndrome, at the time he was the only known patient in the UK to have pulled through.

Alan says: 'One of the worst things was my eyesight being affected so I couldn't drive, I had to give up my licence. Other than that I now swim regularly with a disabled swimming club, I have a part-time job working from home and my health is as good as ever. I truly am a lucky man!'

13

Tests and Treatment

As I have said repeatedly throughout this book the key to tackling Hughes syndrome is getting a diagnosis. The most fundamental way to achieve this is to have the blood tests specifically designed to detect antibodies linked to the illness. If you suspect you have 'sticky blood' then ask to be tested. It costs little and will either put your mind at rest or confirm your fears and help you to the next stage, which is getting treatment.

There are two tests being used at the moment and they are both widely available in major clinics across the world. You don't have to understand the science behind them, what is important is you remember the names of the tests so you can insist on having them if you wish. There are two tests because there are slight differences between them and some patients may show positive on one and not on the other. To eliminate that gap it is usual to carry out both.

Anticardiolipin antibodies

This is an inexpensive test and is so common it has become standardized in many laboratories worldwide. Labs use special kits that have been developed to speed up the process of analysis.

The laboratory will separate the blood, and place a drop of serum on a glass slide that contains protein and phospholipid. What it then does is measure the actual antibody levels; most labs use anticardiolipin antibodies (aCL) as the standard blood screen.

Lupus anticoagulant

First of all the name is misleading, this is not a test for lupus. Lupus anticoagulant was first identified half a century ago and is a complex blood clotting test. Those working with 'sticky blood' say the test is less reliable than the one for anticardiolipin antibodies and it is more prone to variations between laboratories. But until a replacement test is found, doctors cannot take the risk of avoiding doing this test just in case it comes back positive.

Usually one positive result will not be enough to confirm a diagnosis. Patients are asked to come back after six weeks and be retested. It is odd but it can happen someone is positive the first time and negative the second. No one is sure why this happens but the experts in this field also look for clinical indications of the condition.

If you test positive you will be told your anticardiolipin levels are low, medium or high. The higher the level the more risk there is of thrombosis.

INR

These letters stand for international normalized ratio. It is this measurement that is used to compare the thickness of a patient's blood with what normal blood would measure. The higher the ratio, or INR, the thinner the blood. Most patients feel well with an INR of between 2.0 and 3.0. Some need it to be even thinner and are happiest with an INR of 3.5 to 4.0. Most people have to go to hospital for blood tests but there are self-test machines available enabling a patient to keep an eye on their INR at home. These machines are extremely useful but unfortunately they are also expensive.

Clinical clues

When you see a specialist who knows about Hughes syndrome they will be looking beyond blood tests. The tests can fluctuate between positive and negative. The doctor is looking for physical signs that you have Hughes syndrome. For instance painful joints, eye problems, a medical history of miscarriage or blood-clotting, headaches or strokes. When they examine you they will look for blotchy skin, blue-to-black fingers and toes, and bruising.

Treatment

There is a simple logic to treating Hughes syndrome; the blood is more viscous than it should be, thicker, so the obvious path to go down is to thin the blood. There is one other way of dealing with the condition and that is by trying to suppress the antibodies that cause the problem in the first place, but this is a tricky proposition as it involves interfering with an already abnormal immune system.

Doctors prefer to target the clotting tendency. They prescribe a number of drugs known as 'anticoagulants' that thin the blood. It sounds frightening but the evidence is there are few side-effects with this range of medication, sometimes a patient can bleed heavily but with the right monitoring that can be avoided. The benefits of taking these drugs can be substantial, their effectiveness can be apparent within days, if not hours in some cases.

There are three drugs commonly used. They are aspirin, warfarin and heparin.

Aspirin

The miracle drug of the last century is still working its magic in the new millennium. Aspirin has long been recognized for its ability to make blood platelets less 'sticky'. Well beyond the field of Hughes syndrome aspirin is used for those who have thrombosis, heart attacks or strokes. Low-dose aspirin (75–100 mg/day) is regarded as a brilliant blood thinner with the least side-effects. In rare cases a patient may be allergic to aspirin, but there are other drugs in the pharmaceutical armoury that will also do the job with Hughes syndrome.

In milder cases, taking aspirin shows clear benefits; some patients who have got through a serious episode and are now generally well only need to take aspirin to control their symptoms. One area where aspirin shows its effectiveness is in pregnancy. In the lupus pregnancy clinic at St Thomas' Hospital the addition of aspirin helped improve the success rate dramatically amongst women who had suffered recurrent miscarriage.

Heparin

This is perhaps the least popular treatment of the three as it is administered by injection, usually beneath the skin at the side of the stomach or thigh. Patients often learn how to inject themselves. Doctors tend not to use this treatment over a long period of time. Heparin does have its plus points:

- It is possible to reverse its blood thinning effects quite quickly, which is useful if a patient needs an operation.
- Heparin is safe to use throughout pregnancy whereas warfarin cannot be used.
- Heparin works much more quickly than warfarin, it can take

effect within hours whereas warfarin can take a day or so to kick in.

Warfarin

Warfarin, a coumarin anticoagulant, which is also known in some countries as Coumadin, is the standard treatment for thrombosis. It is widely prescribed to treat strokes and TIAs (transient ischaemic attacks or mini-strokes). This drug has been shown to be highly effective in the long-term treatment of 'sticky blood'. It is relatively free of side-effects and is taken orally as a pill. Once a patient is on this medication he or she must have regular tests to check the thickness of the blood, using the INR.

The correct dose is found by a process of trial and error, the aim is to keep the blood twice or three times as thin as normal depending on the severity of the symptoms.

Alternatives

Many people who discover they have an incurable disease look for alternatives to the hefty regime of medicines they will be on for the rest of their lives. The problem that arises with a relatively 'new' condition like Hughes syndrome is that very little research has been done into what natural products might help. If anything a patient has to be extra cautious because when you are taking warfarin (Coumadin in the USA) there are plenty of herbs and other 'remedies' that are contraindicated, in other words potentially harmful.

Doctors do not specifically recommend any alternatives to the mainstream drugs prescribed to patients. What they do say is people on warfarin should watch their alcohol consumption and only take aspirin under doctor's advice. They also reiterate all the usual health advice to autoimmune sufferers: do not smoke, eat a balanced diet, rest and take exercise when you are able; avoid stress if you can. Some Hughes syndrome patients take vitamin supplements, mainly E and C, for their antioxidant qualities. The team at St Thomas' say a large number of patients take cod liver oil because they feel it has an anti-thrombotic effect.

Talking to a wider sample of people with 'sticky blood' the general feeling was to keep away from alternative medications because of the warfarin and the possibility of affecting the delicate balance of the INR. Some took garlic, echinacea, cod liver oil and aloe vera gel capsules and believed these helped as they acted like anticoagulants. With many natural products it is not always possible to know how much is contained in each pill. Plants naturally can vary in strength and this makes it difficult to know exactly what dose you are taking.

As one woman pointed out, if this were not such a life-threatening illness she would be trying everything in the book but she felt it was just too dangerous to take a chance on the unknown. She had tried many treatments like acupuncture, reflexology, Reiki and aromatherapy; they all made her feel better but unfortunately they cost too much to carry on for any length of time.

If you are considering taking alternative medicines it is important that you tell your physician. It is potentially dangerous to self-medicate. There are qualified alternative practitioners (e.g. homeopaths), some of whom are also doctors. You can ask your GP for a referral.

Contacts and Further Reading

Organizations and Websites

The Hughes Syndrome Foundation

St Thomas' Hospital,
London SE1 7EH
Phone 020 7960 5561
Fax 020 7633 0462
Website: http://www.hughes-syndrome.org

Hughes Syndrome Awareness Week takes place every year from 1 to 7 September.

Antiphospholipid syndrome (UK)

Website: http://groups.yahoo.com

If you search for APLSUK there is an excellent online support group. This leads you to some of the few face-to-face support groups that have been set up. If you sign up for this group and go to the bookmarks section on their page there are lots more links and references. APLSUK is the fun group with light-hearted banter as well as serious discussion.

Website: http://forums.delphiforums.com/apsantibody/start/

A forum where questions are answered by others with APS and there are discussions, debates and support.

Website:
http://www.healthcyclopedia.com/antiphospholipid_syndrome.html

A page in an online encyclopaedia that has lots of links and articles and pages on APS/Hughes syndrome on the web.

Antiphospholipid syndrome (USA)

American Auto-immunity Related Diseases Association
Information on lots of diseases related to APS/sticky blood and it includes articles on APS.
Website: http://www.aarda.org

Website://www.rheumatology.org

This is a website with a list of rheumatologists in the USA. There are no APS/Hughes syndrome clinics as such, so this site is useful for finding doctors who know about this condition.

Lupus UK

St James House,
Eastern Road,
Romford, Essex RM1 3NH
Phone 01708 731251
Fax 01708 731252
Website: http://www.lupusuk.com

The St Thomas' Lupus Trust

St Thomas' Hospital,
London SE1 7EH
Phone 020 7922 8197
Fax 020 7960 5698
Email: sally@lupus.org.uk
Website: http://www.lupus.org.uk

The Migraine Trust

45 Great Ormond Street,
London WC1N 3HZ
Phone: 020 7831 4818
Fax 020 7831 5174
Website: http://www.migrainetrust.org

Brings together support for the benefit of people with headache conditions.

Miscarriage

The Association for Improvement in Maternity Services (AIMS)
Website: http://www.aims.org.uk

Babyloss.com
Babyloss is an exclusively online resource for anyone whose life has been touched by pregnancy loss, stillbirth or neonatal death. They cannot offer medical advice, but will always endeavour to point visitors at the relevant organizations or individuals in order to receive the help required.

The Child Bereavement Trust
The Child Bereavement Trust is a national charity founded to improve the support offered by professionals to grieving families when a baby or child dies and when children experience the death of a mother, father, brother or sister. The charity provides specialized training and support for professionals and also produces resources and information for bereaved children and families.
Website: www.childbereavement.org.uk

The Miscarriage Association
Website: http://www.miscarriageassociation.org.uk

The National Infertility Support Network (CHILD)
Charter House,
43 St Leonards Road,
Bexhill on Sea, East Sussex TN40 1JA
Email: officechild.org.uk

Women's Health Information
Website: http://www.womens-health.co.uk

The Stroke Association

Website: http://www.stroke.org.uk

Stroke Survivors

For survivors of cerebral stroke.
Website: http://www.stroke-survivors.co.uk

Alternative Medicine

The Hale Clinic,
7 Park Crescent,
London W1B 1PF
Phone 020 7631 0156
Website: http://www.haleclinic.com

Further Reading

Dr Graham Hughes, *Hughes Syndrome: Patient's Guide*, Springer, 2001.

M. A. Khamashta (ed.), *Hughes Syndrome: Antiphospholipid Syndrome*, Springer, 2000.
A clinical and scientific guide, for doctors and researchers, with contributions from 57 of the world's leading authorities.

Index